ANXIETY AND DEPRESSION:

YOUR QUESTIONS ANSWERED

D1362738

For Churchill Livingstone

Publisher Timothy Horne
Project Editor Jane Shanks
Project Controller Nancy Arnott
Design Direction Erik Bigland

ANXIETY AND DEPRESSION:
YOUR QUESTIONS ANSWERED

Cosmo Hallstrom

MB ChB MD (Liverpool) MRCP (UK) FRCPsych

Formerly Consultant Psychiatrist, Charing Cross Hospital; Medical Director, Charter Clinic, Chelsea; Senior Lecturer, Institute of Psychiatry and Imperial College Medical School;

Nicola McClure

MBBS MRCGP

Principal in General Practice, Shepherds Bush, London

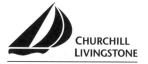

CHURCHILL
LIVINGSTONE

EDINBURGH LONDON NEW YORK PHILADELPHIA SYDNEY TORONTO 1998

CHURCHILL LIVINGSTONE
An imprint of Harcourt Publishers Limited

Robert Stevenson House, 1–3 Baxter's Place, Leith Walk,
Edinburgh EH1 3AF, UK

First published 1998
  Reprinted 2000

ISBN 0 443 04939 4

British Library of Cataloguing in Publication Data
A catalogue record for this book is available from the
British Library.

Library of Congress Cataloging in Publication Data
A catalog record for this book is available from the Library
of Congress.

Medical knowledge is constantly changing. As information
becomes available, changes in treatment, procedures,
equipment and the use of drugs become necessary. The
authors and publishers have, as far as it is possible, taken
care to ensure that the information given in the text is
accurate and up to date. However, readers are strongly
advised to confirm that the information, especially with
regard to drug usage, complies with current legislation and
standards of practice.

The
publisher's
policy is to use
**paper manufactured
from sustainable forests**

Printed in China
GCC/02

CONTENTS

INTRODUCTION

As anxiety and depression are among the commonest of conditions that GPs will encounter, their care is increasingly being devolved to primary care. With modern treatments, both medical and psychological, we are now able to offer patients more, and there is increasing awareness of the depth of the conditions and of the value of early and intensive treatment to prevent chronicity. Indeed these are very treatable conditions.

This book follows a simple question and answer format. It is not a standard textbook on the subject but offers a dialogue between the GP and psychiatrist, who have had a long working relationship. It hopes to offer practical advice on real clinical problems as encountered on a daily basis. Much of it will be advice that is not found in standard textbooks, and which is intended to continue where they leave off.

The book is aimed primarily at GPs who are involved in the daily care of anxious and depressed patients. It should also be of value to community psychiatric nurses, psychologists and social workers to enable them to understand the thinking that goes on in the management of depressed patients and hopefully takes them forward as well in their daily management of patients with anxiety and depression. It should also be of value to patients and their families, helping to unravel some of the medical mystique that may surround their problem and its treatment. It should enable them to become more involved in their treatment, thereby reaching a more rapid and effective resolution.

ABBREVIATIONS USED IN THIS BOOK

5-HT	5-hydroxytryptamine
CNS	central nervous system
CSM	Committee on the Safety of Medicines
DSM4	Diagnostic and Statistical Manual of the American Medical Association 4
ECG	electrocardiogram
ECT	electroconvulsive therapy
EEG	electroencephalogram
ENT	ear, nose and throat
GABA	gamma amino butyric acid
GABA-B	gamma amino butyric acid-B
HADS	Hospital Anxiety and Depression Scale
HAMD	Hamilton Depression Rating Scale
HRT	hormone replacement therapy
IBS	irritable bowel syndrome
ICD10	International Classification of Diseases 10 edition
MAO	monoamine oxidase
MAO-A	monoamine oxidase-A
MAOI	monoamine oxidase inhibitor
ME	myalgic encephalomyelitis
MHPG	3-methoxy-4-hydroxyphenylglycol
NaSSA	noradrenergic and specific serotonergic antidepressant
OCD	obsessive compulsive disorder
PMT	premenstrual tension
RIMA	reversible monoamine oxidase inhibitor
SAD	seasonal affective disorder
SNRI	serotonin noradrenergic reuptake inhibitors
SSRI	selective serotonin (5-hydroxytryptamine) reuptake inhibitors

THE DIAGNOSIS OF ANXIETY

Introduction

Anxiety is characterized by unrealistic or excessive worry about life circumstances and a series of physical symptoms which persist for a period of some weeks and are present on most days. The prime consideration is the level of severity and functional impairment that this and other key symptoms cause, since most people have minor transient symptoms from time to time which require no intervention. Those patients who have severe and disabling symptoms certainly require treatment.

1.1

How is anxiety classified?

There are currently two major classification systems. The International Classification of Diseases (ICD10) and the Diagnostic and Statistical Manual of the American Psychiatric Association (DSM4). The DSM4 is designed to provide operational criteria to enable patients to be diagnosed accurately and reliably. Diagnoses should have some clinical relevance in relation to syndrome specificity and prognosis. The DSM4 has strict operational criteria so that if patients fulfil certain clusters of symptoms in the absence of others they have a defined diagnosis. The ICD10 uses diagnostic criteria more acceptable to ordinary European clinical descriptions offering broad outlines of syndromes.

The main diagnostic groups of the ICD10 and DSM4 are shown in Table 1. In the absence of biological markers, these criteria are derived from clinical descriptions. As well as the clinical syndromes, the DSM4 system includes secondary classifications describing developmental and personality disorders, physical disorders, the severity of psychosocial stresses and a global assessment of functioning. Thus, this

Table 1.1 DSM4 (World Health Organization 1992, Geneva) and ICD10 (American Psychiatric Association 1994, Washington) Diagnostic categories of some anxiety disorders

DSM4	ICD10
Panic disorder without agoraphobia	Panic disorder
Generalized anxiety disorder	Generalized anxiety disorder
Panic with agoraphobia	Agoraphobia with panic
Agoraphobia without panic	Agoraphobia without panic
Social phobia	Social phobia
Specific phobia	Specific phobia
Obsessive compulsive disorder	Obsessive compulsive disorder
Post-traumatic stress disorder	Post-traumatic stress disorder
	Mixed anxiety and depression
	Neurasthenia
	Depersonalization–derealization syndrome
Somatization syndrome	Somatoform disorder
Acute stress disorder	

system takes into account not only the diagnosis, but related causal factors and severity.

1.2

Is it necessary to adopt rigid diagnostic criteria in general practice?

It is unusual to see the full syndrome in clinical practice. The problem with being too precise in diagnosis is that it excludes the common fact that most patients fulfil more than one diagnostic criterion, and often shift from one diagnosis to another. The systems are not perfect. However, for the time being they offer us the best system available.

1.3

Do rigid diagnostic criteria have any relevance to treatment?

There appear to be distinct differences between the major clinical syndromes, and this can affect both treatment and outcome, and at that point diagnosis becomes clinically relevant to the GP. For example, panic disorder is best treated with either cognitive therapy and reassurance, or antidepressants. Generalized anxiety disorder probably responds best to relaxation training or buspirone. Obsessive compulsive disorder (OCD) probably has a different causation to other anxiety disorders, and antidepressants would probably be a first-line treatment, especially the 5-hydroxytryptamine (5-HT) selective serotonin reuptake inhibitors (SSRIs), in addition to behaviour therapy. Social phobias probably respond best to systematic desensitization or antidepressants, and post-traumatic stress disorder to sedation and brief focused psychotherapy.

1.4

Is there a reliable instrument for assessing anxiety that I can use in the surgery?

The severity of an anxiety state can be determined by the number of symptoms the patient has and the level of functional impairment. The

3

best instrument for measuring anxiety in a practice situation is the Hospital Anxiety and Depression Scale (HADS), which also helps distinguish between anxiety and depression. It is a simple 14-question scale designed for self-rating inpatients who may also have physical problems (Fig. 1.1). A score of 0 to 7 is no clinical anxiety, 8 to 10 is borderline, 11 to 16 is moderate and 17 to 24 is severe. Treatment should be considered with a score of 15 or more (Fig. 1.1).

The well-known Hamilton Depression Rating Scale (HAMD) is an observer rating scale, to be completed by the GP. This is useful but more time-consuming (Fig. 1.2). It is probably appropriate to treat patients who score 15 or more.

1.5

Can these scales be used repeatedly to assess improvement after treatment?

Rating scales are useful in establishing the severity and breadth of the clinical syndrome, and even more so for measuring and detecting change as patients improve as a result of treatment. They can be applied repeatedly with the proviso that the patient should only rate the way they have felt over the preceding 3 days. They are useful in enabling the patient, as well as the doctor, to monitor progress.

It is sometimes useful to ask patients to draw up their own rating scale of key items which they can chart daily on a three-point scale from absent to severe. This demystifies symptoms and introduces the idea that not all symptoms are permanent and immutable, but subject to change over time and often in response to environmental factors.

1.6

At what stage does normal anxiety become pathological?

There is no clear demarcation point where normal anxiety becomes pathological and should be treated. Basically, when anxiety is unrealistic and excessive, it can be regarded as pathological. It warrants treatment when it interferes with normal living and when it is felt to be distressing and persistent. Ultimately, it is reducible to a value judgement: when the patient seeks help, the clinician has to

Doctors are aware that emotions play an important part in most illnesses. If your doctor knows about these feelings, he/she will be able to help you more.

This questionnaire is designed to help your doctor to know how you feel. Read each item and circle the score beside the reply which comes closest to how you have been feeling in the past week.

Don't take too long over your replies; your immediate reaction to each item will probably be more accurate than a long thought out response.

Circle one score per item

D / A		D / A	
	I feel tense or 'wound up':		*I feel as if I am slowed down:*
3	Most of the time	3	Nearly all the time
2	A lot of the time	2	Very often
1	From time to time, occasionally	1	Sometimes
0	Not at all	0	Not at all
	I still enjoy the things I used to enjoy:		*I get a sort of frightened feeling like 'butterflies' in the stomach:*
0	Definitely as much		
1	Not quite so much	0	Not at all
2	Only a little	1	Occasionally
3	Hardly at all	2	Quite often
		3	Very often
	I get a sort of frightened feeling as if something awful is about to happen:		*I have lost interest in my appearance:*
3	Very definitely and quite badly	3	Definitely
2	Not quite so much now	2	I don't take so much care as I should
1	Definitely not so much now	1	I may not take quite as much care
0	Not at all	0	I take just as much care as ever
	I can laugh and see the funny side of things:		*I feel restless as if I have to be on the move:*
0	As much as I always could	3	Very much indeed
1	Not quite so much now	2	Quite a lot
2	Definitely not so much now	1	Not very much
3	Not at all	0	Not at all
	Worrying thoughts go through my mind:		*I look forward with enjoyment to things:*
3	A great deal of the time	0	As much as I ever did
2	A lot of the time	1	Rather less than I used to
1	From time to time but not too often	2	Definitely less than I used to
0	Only occasionally	3	Hardly at all
	I feel cheerful:		*I get sudden feelings of panic:*
3	Not at all	3	Very often indeed
2	Not often	2	Quite often
1	Sometimes	1	Not very often
0	Most of the time	0	Not at all
	I can sit at ease and feel relaxed:		*I can enjoy a good book or radio or TV programme:*
0	Definitely	0	Often
1	Usually	1	Sometimes
2	Not often	2	Not often
3	Not at all	3	Very seldom

Now check to be sure you have answered all the questions

Total score and grading

Total score: Anxiety _____ Depression _____

Grading: 0–7 Non case   8–10 Borderline case   11+ Case

Fig. 1.1 Hospital Anxiety and Depression Scale (HADS) which is completed by the patient. The scoring system has been added to the questionnaire. (From Zigmond AS, Snaith RP 1983. The hospital anxiety and depression scale. Acta Psychiatrica Scandinavica 67:361–370.)

Please grade response as assessed over the past 7 days as 0 – 4 using the scale below:

0 = Not present
1 = Mild
2 = Moderate
3 = Severe
4 = Very severe (grossly disabling)

Anxious mood
Worries, anticipation of the worst, fearful anticipation, irritability.

Tension
Feelings of tension, fatiguability, startle response, moved to tears easily, trembling, feelings of restlessness, inability to relax.

Fears
Of dark, of strangers, of being left alone, of animals, of traffic, of crowds.

Insomnia
Difficulty in falling asleep, broken sleep, unsatisfying sleep and fatigue on waking, dreams nightmares, night terrors. *Add 1 point if the patient is taking night sedation.*

Intellectual
Difficulty in concentrating, poor memory.

Depressed mood
Loss of interest, lack of pleasure in hobbies, depression, early waking, diurnal swing.

Somatic (muscular)
Pains and aches, twitchings, stiffness, myoclonic jerks, grinding teeth, unsteady voice.

Somatic (sensory)
Tinnitus, blurring of vision, hot and cold flushes, feelings of weakness, prickling sensation.

Cardiovascular symptoms
Tachycardia, palpitations, pain in the chest, throbbing of vessels, fainting feelings, missing beat.

Respiratory symptoms
Pressure or constriction in chest, choking feelings, sighing, dyspnoea.

Gastrointestinal symptoms
Difficulty in swallowing, wind, abdominal pain, burning sensations, abdominal fullness, waterbrash, nausea, vomiting, sinking feelings, 'working' in abdomen, borborygmi, looseness of bowels, loss of weight, constipation.

Genitourinary symptoms
Frequency of micturation, urgency of micturation, amenorrhea, menorrhagia, development of frigidity, premature ejaculation, loss of erection, impotence.

Autonomic symptoms
Dry mouth, flushing, pallor, tendency to sweat, giddiness, tension headache, raising of hair.

Behaviour at interview (general)
Tense, fidgeting, restlessness or pacing, tremor of hands, furrowed brow, strained face, increased muscular tone, sighing or rapid respiration, facial pallor.

Behaviour (physiological)
Swallowing, belching, high resting pulse rate, respiration rate over 20/min, brisk tendon jerks, tremor, dilated pupils, exophthalmos, sweating, eyelid twitching.

TOTAL SCORE *(By adding up values in shadowed boxes only)*

Scoring

Under 8	Normal
9 – 15	Mild
16 – 25	Moderate
Over 26	Severe

decide on what level of help is appropriate. In the milder forms of illness, simply listening to the patient's worries can be of immense therapeutic benefit, and one or two 15-minute sessions may well be all that is required. If this is not sufficient, and the symptoms are more troublesome, then you might consider some anxiolytic medication. Treatment should be considered if anxiety rates a score of 15 or higher on the HADS (Fig. 1.1) or the HAMD (Fig. 1.2).

1.7

What is the difference between free-floating anxiety and a specific anxiety disorder?

The term free-floating anxiety was originally used to describe a non-specific anxiety for which no situational or causative explanation could readily be found (an endogenous anxiety). It constituted a ragbag of disorders. Specific anxiety disorder – fear of a particular object – is a phobia.

1.8

What is the relevance of the distinction?

The better the understanding of the types and causes of the condition, the better the provision of treatment.

Generalized anxiety is best treated by relaxation training and learning an approach to overcome and minimize symptoms. Drug therapy with antidepressants or buspirone has a greater part to play in this condition.

If the object of anxiety can be identified, the treatment will be directed at gradually overcoming the fear, by a process of systematic desensitization.

Fig. 1.2 Hamilton Depression Rating Scale (HAMD). To be completed by the doctor. (From Hamilton M 1959. The assessment of anxiety states by rating. British Journal of Medical Psychology 32:50–55.)

1.9

Can the symptoms of anxiety feature in other psychiatric disorders?

There is a fundamental premise in psychiatry which posits a hierarchy of disorders, ranging from organic syndromes at the top to personality disturbances at the bottom. Lower-order conditions are always seen as subservient to higher-order ones, and thus anxiety may be a feature of all the other conditions above it in the hierarchy (Fig. 1.3).

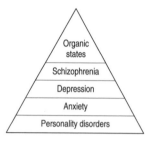

Fig. 1.3 The hierarchy of psychiatric disorders (Laslow).

1.10

What are the main core symptoms of anxiety?

Key symptoms can be classified under the headings of motor tension, autonomic hyperactivity, vigilance and scanning, and, according to the DSM4 classification, six of the 18 symptoms listed in Box 1.1 should be present to make a full diagnosis.

Box 1.1   CORE SYMPTOMS OF ANXIETY

Motor tension
1. Trembling, twitching or feeling shaky
2. Muscle tension, aches or soreness
3. Restlessness
4. Easy fatiguability

Box 1.1   CORE SYMPTOMS OF ANXIETY *CONT'D*

Autonomic hyperactivity
5. Shortness of breath or smothering sensation
6. Palpitations or accelerated heart rate
7. Sweating or cold clammy hands
8. Dry mouth
9. Dizziness or light-headedness
10. Nausea, diarrhoea or other abdominal distress
11. Flushes or hot chills
12. Frequent urination
13. Trouble swallowing or lump in throat

Vigilance and scanning
14. Feeling keyed up or on edge
15. Exaggerated startle response
16. Difficulty concentrating or mind going blank because of anxiety
17. Trouble falling or staying asleep
18. Irritability

It is important to exclude organic pathology, especially thyrotoxicosis, as well as excess caffeine consumption and alcohol or stimulant abuse.

1.11

How are the symptoms of anxiety produced?

Symptoms are generated by physiological and psychological factors.

Box 1.2   MECHANISMS FOR SYMPTOMS OF ANXIETY

Mood
• Fearful apprehension

Thoughts
• Worry

Hyperarousal
• Sleeplessness
• Muscle tension
• Startle response

Somatic
• Sympathetic
• Parasympathetic

Chest
• Hyperventilation
• Palpitations

1.12
What are the common physical symptoms of anxiety disorders?

Somatic symptoms of anxiety mediated by the sympathetic and parasympathetic nervous systems include sweating, diarrhoea, premature ejaculation, palpitations, gastrointestinal disturbances and hyperacidity, dry mouth, nausea and vomiting. Symptoms attributable to hyperarousal include muscle tension which can result in backache, tension headaches and, over a prolonged period of time, temporomandibular arthritis. Hyperventilation can give rise to paraesthesia and chronic fatigue. The list of symptoms is almost endless. While it is hard to extrapolate from one symptom to an underlying anxiety disorder, it is relatively straightforward to see a constellation of symptoms as mediated by an underlying anxiety disorder.

1.13
When physical symptoms of anxiety are prominent, how can one be sure of the diagnosis?

Physical symptoms of anxiety, such as palpitations and arrhythmias, or bowel disturbances, can be difficult to diagnose as part of the anxiety spectrum: even if the psychological symptoms of anxiety are present, it may be difficult to see whether they are secondary or primary to the underlying apparent physical condition. Somatic and psychic symptoms often co-exist, but patients presenting with isolated physical symptoms can be notoriously difficult to diagnose, and are often investigated exhaustively before a negative diagnosis of physical disorder suggests a psychological mechanism. Patients rarely fulfil clear diagnostic criteria for anxiety or depressive disorders, and may seem to fall into a diagnostic no-man's land.

1.14
What are the common physical disorders which may mimic anxiety?

Hyperthyroidism is the only common condition to mimic anxiety. Phaeochromocytomas, idiopathic hypoglycaemia, carcinoid syndrome as well as temporal lobe epilepsy are rare conditions which may also mimic anxiety. The way to approach the problem is to consider alternative pathology if the presentation of the anxiety disorder is atypical. A detailed history should be taken to try to elicit disturbance in other organ systems, or the patient can be referred to a physician. However, hyperthyroidism is simple to exclude and easy to miss, and patients who have panic disorders may present with arrhythmias of uncertain significance. Excess alcohol use and subsequent withdrawal can result in anxiety symptoms as can the abuse of stimulants, such as caffeine overdose, especially in the elderly who lose their tolerance. Labyrinthine disorders should also be considered as a variant of panic disorder.

1.15

Should all patients who present with symptoms of anxiety have their thyroid function tested?

Thyrotoxicosis is the one commonly occurring condition that needs to be excluded; it is easy to test for and rewarding to treat. It probably is not worth testing every patient with anxiety symptoms, but the diagnosis should be borne in mind as a possibility and excluded at least on clinical grounds, especially in those with tachycardia and warm hands. It should be considered in patients where there is no obvious cause for the symptoms, or where the symptom pattern is slightly unusual, especially in people over the age of 30 where the recent onset of an anxiety disorder should be regarded with suspicion.

1.16

Should an electrocardiogram (ECG) be done on anxious patients who experience palpitations?

ECGs rarely reveal any significant pathology, but they might reveal some minor abnormality. This then leads to the question whether further investigation is required. If there is any real doubt about cardiac pathology, then the patient needs to be investigated properly. The decision has to be taken on clinical grounds. Many anxious patients are found in cardiology clinics where minor conduction abnormalities are detected which are of dubious clinical significance.

Investigating an anxious patient may have a very positive therapeutic aspect in providing reassurance that there is nothing wrong with the heart. On the other hand, it may lead to the treadmill of frequent and irrelevant investigations which detract from the main problem of the underlying panic disorder. For example, one man with panic disorder has now had two coronary angiograms done which were normal and could have been avoided if a proper history had been taken.

Unfortunately, many more patients with treatable anxiety states are missed than patients with treatable cardiac disease, but the former is common, and the latter is regarded as unforgivable.

1.17

Are anxious patients at any greater risk of myocardial infarction or hypertension?

Unfortunately, yes. Patients with panic attacks have an increased incidence of mitral valve prolapse when compared to normal controls, although the significance of this is not clear. They are more likely to have cardiac arrhythmias, which is why so many patients with panic disorder go on to be investigated by cardiologists who, with increasingly sophisticated techniques, are able to diagnose functional abnormalities. Neurotic patients are at increased risk of death, which makes reassurance more difficult. Anxious patients have been found to have increased levels of noradrenaline and adrenaline in their blood, and this may result in chronic vasoconstriction and hypertension. Chronic anxiety does result in raised blood pressure, and this may be one of the underlying mechanisms for the increased cardiac morbidity of anxious patients.

1.18

How are patients managed who present with primarily physical complaints of anxiety?

From a therapeutic point of view, the exclusion of a serious physical disorder should be sufficient to reassure the patient that there is nothing seriously wrong. Anxiety management training should be directed at teaching the patient to cope with the symptoms as well as possible, whether they are physically or psychologically induced.

These management techniques are widely used in pain clinics, for cardiac rehabilitation and for the treatment of functional bowel disorders. Even if there is an organic cause for a symptom, it does not mean that a psychological/psychiatric treatment, whether psychological or pharmacological, is not appropriate. For example, patients with breathlessness due to obstructive airways disease benefit from psychological counselling and simple psychotherapy, and also from anxiolytic medication, providing it does not reduce respiratory drive.

1.19

What sort of history should I elicit from a patient with symptoms of anxiety, and what are the main physical symptoms that I should note?

Key questions to ask would include a family history of psychiatric disorders to indicate a genetic predisposition. Other background factors include an alcohol and drug history to indicate self-medication, and simple questions about pre-morbid personality and the onset of the symptoms, with particular emphasis on precipitating factors and the patient's own assessment of the causation. It is helpful to ask about panic attacks, and, if present, their frequency and what triggers them. It is important to exclude obvious physical causes such as thyrotoxicosis, characterized by warm sweaty hands and a rapid resting pulse rate with weight loss, and also to exclude depression as a prominent symptom. Anxiety symptoms emerging de novo in people over the age of 40 may well be secondary to depressive illness (see Box 1.3).

Box 1.3   CHECKLIST OF QUESTIONS TO CONSIDER IN AN ANXIOUS PATIENT

- Family history
- Alcohol and drugs
- Pre-morbid personality
- Main symptoms
- Precipitants to onset of disorder
- Presence and frequency of panic attacks
- Possible organic causation
- Possible other primary psychiatric disorders, especially depression

---

Non-verbal signs of anxiety disorders include rapid speech, tiredness, sitting on the edge of the chair, an exaggerated startle response, but in general these are relatively non-specific. A moderate tachycardia would also be associated with an anxiety disorder.

1.20
Do any other animals show similar signs of stress?

Animals can be shown to suffer from stress caused, for example, by overcrowding. If stressed too much, lions develop hypertrophy of the adrenal glands. Some animals, usually those preyed upon by others, are naturally anxious. Grazing animals of the savannah or grasslands are much more jumpy and prepared for flight than elephants or predators such as lions. One can demonstrate differing degrees of anxiety in experimental mice strains, which can be bred for high or low anxiety levels.

Mice and rats, as well as higher vertebrates, are used in experimental models of anxiety, especially for drug development. Thus, it is possible to cause stress and anxiety states in animals. Veterinary surgeons also recognize anxiety and depressive states among pets, which often reflect the attitudes of their owners.

1.21
How do other animals cope with stress?

Animals cope with stress in different ways. Stress may be beneficial, incorporating the fight-or-flight response.

Camels, which are able to withstand periods of considerable physical hardship with apparent calm, are known to have high levels of endorphins in the pituitary which may be the mechanism of their physiological tolerance to hardship. Benzodiazepine receptors are found throughout the vertebrate kingdom, and even in invertebrates, such as lobsters, in a modified form. Presumably, these receptors are related to the mechanism controlling arousal.

Stress may also be destructive, resulting in maladaptive behaviour and physical deterioration. Monkeys become aggressive and self-destructive, for example, picking at their skin and becoming apathetic and withdrawn.

1.22

How are anxiety and stress differentiated?

Anxiety is a generalized pervasive fear associated with apprehension and worry and with the avoidance of frightening situations. There is a constellation of subjective symptoms and behaviour, resulting in a syndrome which may be regarded as an illness, or at least as pathological. Stress is the external force which results in the symptoms of anxiety. The definitions tend to be used rather loosely. Whereas anxiety is considered to be an illness, stress is somewhat less prejudicial and is seen as an individual's appropriate response to definable external problems, such as pressure of work or battle. Diagnosis of stress-related disorders is increasingly common, and eliminates the stigma of mental illness. Stress clinics and stress counsellors are gaining in acceptability, especially in the business world. Stress management is discussed in Chapter 8.

1.23

I have found that patients often prefer me to write stress or anxiety on their certificates rather than depression. Do you feel that there is still considerable stigma attached to depression whilst the concept of stress and anxiety has become more acceptable?

Unfortunately one of the major bars to patients accepting treatment is the problem of stigma. We are forever inventing new euphemisms to deal with stigma until the euphemism becomes common parlance and a new euphemism needs to be developed. In my experience when most people acknowledge that they have a depressive illness or emotional problems they receive a lot of support from their peers who will also admit to having had problems in the past.

1.24

Why are some people more prone to developing anxiety and stress symptoms than others?

There is a clear genetic basis to anxiety disorders. Some people are born more anxious than others.

People learn to cope with stress by dealing properly with anxiety-provoking situations. If dealt with badly, similar situations arising in the future will be met with fear. For example, if children feel threatened and abandoned in childhood, as adults they will find situations which remind them of those feelings more threatening than will those who have had a more secure upbringing.

Neurotic (self-destructive) ways of dealing with anxiety are also learned. Children with anxious parents are more likely to develop maladaptive ways of behaving by modelling themselves on their parents.

People who have learned to be secure within themselves are better able to cope with stresses as they arise than people who have learned poor ways of coping with anxiety-provoking situations.

On top of this comes the personal meaning of the anxiety-provoking situation to the individual, and his or her attitude to life in general. For example, the threat of redundancy would be far more anxiety provoking to a middle-aged man with a mortgage and family to support than to a young man who was not happy in his job and was thinking of changing work for employment with better prospects.

Within the anxiety spectrum are found conditions such as alcoholism and drug abuse which may have developed because of underlying anxiety traits.

There are genetic, biological, developmental and environmental factors which contribute to the development of anxiety disorders. The problem lies in determining the way they interact and the relative influence of each factor. At present, the answer depends to a great extent on the approach taken by the person posing the question. Special groups are dealt with in Chapter 5.

1.25

Why do some people thrive on anxiety and others suffer from it?

Anxiety has two components: 'trait', which is an underlying predisposition to the level of anxiety the individual has as a baseline; and 'state', which is a variable function depending upon external factors. Most individuals have an optimal anxiety or arousal level at which they feel and function best.

People with low basal anxiety often seek anxiety-provoking situations such as dangerous sports and are generally regarded as thrill-seekers. Other people with high anxiety levels tend to try to reduce their anxiety by avoiding situations that increase anxiety.

1.26

What is the best approach to treating severe anxiety?

Some people suffer chronically from such disabling anxiety that it prevents them from living a normal life, and this degree of anxiety is extremely difficult to treat. Referral to a specialist would be appropriate when all the options available to a GP have been exhausted. Specialists could offer more intensive pharmacotherapy, such as monoamine oxidase inhibitors (MAOIs) and a wide range of other antidepressants. More structured psychological therapies may be appropriate from a clinical psychologist, or attendance at a day hospital could provide structure and a way of channelling anxieties in a more positive direction. In extreme circumstances inpatient admission may be appropriate, with a period of sedation, which at least provides a temporary respite. In intractable cases, there is the possibility of psychosurgery, although this is very rarely performed these days.

Anxiety disorders may be intractable in some individuals. Some patients, because of a mixture of anxiety symptoms, domestic circumstances and personality factors, may make themselves incurable. In such cases a strategy of providing as many supports as possible in the form of community psychiatric nurses and attendance at day centres should be pursued to offer as much social relief as possible.

1.27

What is the role of neurotransmitters in anxiety and its treatment?

Noradrenaline appears to be involved in the mechanism of anxiety since episodes of increased anxiety, especially with panic attacks, are associated with marked peripheral sympathetic activation because of excessive noradrenaline release. Elevated levels of 3-methoxy-4-hydroxyphenylglycol (MHPG), a metabolite of noradrenaline, have been found in anxiety. Also, the locus ceruleus (rich in noradrenergic fibres), when stimulated in animals, can produce signs of arousal that strongly resemble those seen in human anxiety states. These mechanisms appear to offer one explanation for the mechanism of panic attacks. 5-hydroxytryptamine (serotonin or 5-HT) is also involved in the mechanism of anxiety, although exactly how is unclear. It is made more complex by the large number of 5-HT receptor subtypes (seven now identified). The benzodiazepine receptor coupled to the gamma amino butyric acid (GABA) receptor complex is also involved in anxiety regulation since benzodiazepines are such effective anxiolytics, but the natural benzodiazepine is not yet identified. Other anxiogenic peptides are also involved including cholecystokinin and opioids. Buspirone and other drugs acting on $5-HT_{1a}$ receptors are effective anxiolytics. Selective serotonin reuptake inhibitor (SSRI) antidepressants also appear to be effective antidepressants, as well as being good for panic and OCDs. The fact that antidepressants which only block noradrenaline do not appear to be effective in anxiety and panic disorder mediates against the involvement of noradrenaline. There is, unfortunately, a large gap between theory and practice, and it is likely that more than one mechanism is involved in the regulation of anxiety in each individual and that one may exert control over another further down the neuronal line.

2 THE DIAGNOSIS OF DEPRESSION

Introduction

The concept of melancholia (black bile) was mentioned in texts of Hippocrates. Since then the somatic element of mental illness has vied with the theological interpretation of melancholy as a consequence of sin. In the 18th and 19th centuries, concepts of melancholy concentrated on the symptomatology rather than the causation, and around this period, humane treatments and attitudes to insanity began to develop.

The modern concepts of depression evolved towards the end of the 19th century, when depressive illnesses were seen as distinct from other forms of mental illness such as schizophrenia and general paralysis of the insane. The modern classifications derive from this, although concentrating on the severe end of the spectrum. The final stage in the recognition of depressive disorders has come about since the Second World War as a result of a liberalizing of society and increased access to health care. More importantly, the application of electroconvulsive therapy (ECT) to depression and the development of effective antidepressants made it a worthwhile task to seek out patients with depression.

Thus, after the introduction of imipramine in 1957 and of the MAOI isoniazid in 1958, treatment became available for patients who previously had spent prolonged periods in mental hospitals. The success with the more severe end of the spectrum encouraged treatment of patients with the less severe disorders. The development of antidepressants with less debilitating side effects, increasing access to information and patient expectations have resulted in greater awareness, recognition and treatment of depression. More recently, there has been increasing interest in the social and psychological antecedents of depressive illness.

2.1

Are the terms endogenous or exogenous (reactive) still used to describe depression?

This classification relies upon supposed causation of the illness, where exogenous or reactive depression is seen as arising out of circumstances bearing upon the individual, and endogenous or biological depression is thought to arise without obvious precipitant. In general, exogenous depression was seen as less severe, and endogenous more severe. These conditions are now understood to be more complicated in their causation, and more complex models are used. For example, life events (bereavement, unemployment, moving house and the break-up of relationships) can act as triggers to what would previously have been seen as a biological or severe type of depression. Equally, some people who encounter adversity in their life get depressed while others seem to cope with all circumstances.

2.2

Does this classification have any significance for treatment or prognosis of depression?

External precipitating factors are relevant to the understanding of the condition and its management, but should not preclude diagnosis or treatment. Regarding prognosis, if considerable stresses are acting upon individuals, it must be more difficult to treat the illness biologically even though a biological mechanism underlies the ability to withstand stress.

The decision to treat is more dependent upon the severity of the illness than its causation. Antidepressants tend not to work in milder depression and appear effective in severe depression whatever the cause. Psychological therapies are less effective at the severe end of the spectrum.

2.3

What is major depression?

The standard diagnostic criteria require at least five of the symptoms in Box 2.1 to be present during the same 2-week period, representing a change from previous functioning in the absence of an organic cause, bereavement reaction or other major mental illness. One of the first two must be present.

Box 2.1   DIAGNOSTIC CRITERIA FOR MAJOR DEPRESSION
1. Depressed mood 2. Loss of interest or pleasure 3. Significant weight loss 4. Insomnia or hypersomnia 5. Psychomotor agitation or retardation 6. Fatigue or loss of interest 7. Feelings of worthlessness or guilt 8. Poor concentration 9. Recurrent thoughts of death

2.4

What is the peak age for a depressive illness?

The high prevalence rates are found in the 18- to 30-year-olds. Rates drop with increasing age. It appears that depression is becoming more common, and this probably reflects a true increase, rather than better recognition. The increase is probably due to psychosocial factors such as altered expectations rather than biological factors.

2.5

Is there a genetic basis for depression?

A strong genetic basis for the inheritance of severe depressive illnesses has been demonstrated in the study of twins, where identical twins separated at birth have a high concordance for depression. Risk factors for depression are about 10% if one parent has a history, and greater if both parents are affected. As a clinician, I often see depression commonly running in families where a parent, grandparent or uncle or aunt also have the illness.

2.6

To what extent can depression be considered a learned behaviour?

An element of learned behaviour is involved; inheritance is not sufficient to account for all cases of depression. There is an interaction between nature and nurture, although the more I see, the more I believe in genetic influences as having a strong part to play.

2.7

What is the biochemical basis of depression?

If only we knew! The amine hypothesis of depression suggests that there are functional deficiencies of the neurotransmitters 5-HT, dopamine and noradrenaline, but this is now regarded as too simplistic a view. Reduced levels of dopamine may be the mechanism for reduced psychomotor activity in depression and elevated activity in mania. Acetylcholine may also be involved, but it has not yet been studied thoroughly. These neurotransmitters work in the synapse between nerve cells. There is considerable interest in second messenger systems which act after the receptor and generate further nerve impulses. Because of the complex nature of the nervous system, where one neurotransmitter system closely interacts with another, it is impossible to say where the primary disturbance lies, and to disentangle what is a primary phenomenon, and what is a secondary effect in the control of mood.

2.8

Is there a relationship between food and depression?

The relationship between food and mood regulation is only partially understood. Chocolate, for example, contains phenylethylamine, an indirectly acting sympathomimetic which causes the release of noradrenaline. Theoretically, this could then increase noradrenaline neurotransmission and act as an antidepressant. Phenylethylamine, however, is inactivated in the liver by monoamine oxidases (MAOs), so unless a person is taking an MAOI, only minute amounts will get into the systemic circulation. Nevertheless, chocolate eating can precipitate migraine, probably through the phenylethylamine effect. Chocolate also contains theobromine, a caffeine-like alkaloid, which may have mood enhancing properties. Meat and other proteins contain L-tryptophan, a precursor of 5-HT, another neurotransmitter implicated in depression. L-tryptophan given in doses of a gram a day appears to have an antidepressant effect. Unfortunately, commercially produced L-tryptophan is subject to close control because eosinophilias have resulted from impurities in the manufacture of the substance. To get enough L-tryptophan from a normal diet one would have to eat several pounds of steak per day. Food and glucose can have an effect upon mood, as hunger increases vigilance and irritability, and the consumption of a large meal gives feelings of well being, drowsiness and sluggishness. This has been attributed to a diversion of the blood supply away from the brain and to the stomach. However, it is more likely to be a result of the blood glucose levels and other more complex neuro-humoral regulatory systems.

Mood and eating are closely linked. A subtype of depression, more prevalent among young women, is characterized by binge eating, where patients initially derive emotional satisfaction from bingeing; patients with this disorder respond well to MAOIs. The control of appetite is mediated by 5-HT and dopaminergic systems in the hypothalamus. Amphetamines act as appetite suppressants and also euphoriants. There are also psychological cues related to eating, especially 'naughty but nice' foodstuffs such as chocolate.

2.9

Is depression more common in the winter when it is cold and dark?

Severe depression, as reflected by admission to mental hospital, is commoner in spring and summer, as is suicide, although there is a peak incidence for manic depressive illness in the autumn. Peaks in suicide rates occur in the southern hemisphere in November (spring). The reason for this is not clear. It has been suggested that the depressed individual feels more alienated at a time when nature is undergoing rebirth. Equally, increasing light can affect pineal hormones, complex compounds which may contain within them neurotransmitters. Another view is that seasonal depression is a variant of hibernation, although the statistical relationship is weak. It is not uncommon for people to feel mildly depressed as the hours of darkness increase. Regular depressive episodes may appear for a period of some months in regular cycles every year. This is called Seasonal Affective Disorder (SAD).

Some affective disorders peak in the autumn. Some are followed by a period of hypomania. Depressive phases usually start when hours of daylight diminish after summer and tend to last for about 4 months. It is about six times as common in women than men. There is a direct correlation between latitude and the incidence of SAD, which is higher among the population living north of the Arctic Circle, and seems to fall in the population living nearer the Equator.

2.10
What is the Hamilton Depression Rating Scale?

This scale, devised by Max Hamilton in the late 1950s and the most widely used depression rating scale in the world, assumes that the more symptoms you have and the worse they are, the worse the depression is. Despite its limitations, it has stood the test of time. It is used to detect change more than an absolute measure of severity and is to be filled out by the doctor. A score of 0 to 7 is normal, 8 to 17 mild depression, 18 to 25 moderate and over 26 is severe (Fig. 2.1, abbreviated version).

2.11
What are the core symptoms of depression?

These are symptoms which most closely identify the illness, and are the ones most likely to change as a result of treatment (see Box 2.2). If three of these are present, then the patient is probably depressed; the presence of four or more should result in a treatment programme.

Hamilton Depression Rating Scale

Patient Name: Date:

	SCORE RANGE	SCORE
1. Depressed mood	0 – 4	
2. Guilt	0 – 4	
3. Suicide	0 – 4	
4. Insomnia – early	0 – 2	
5. Insomnia – middle	0 – 2	
6. Insomnia – late	0 – 2	
7. Work and activities	0 – 4	
8. Retardation	0 – 4	
9. Agitation	0 – 4	
10. Anxiety psychic	0 – 4	
11. Anxiety somatic	0 – 4	
12. Somatic symptoms: gastrointestinal	0 – 2	
13. Somatic symptoms: general	0 – 2	
14. Genital symptoms	0 – 2	
15. Hypochondriasis	0 – 4	
16. Loss of weight	0 – 2	
17. Insight	0 – 2	
TOTAL SCORE		

Score Interpretation Guide:

0 – 7	None/minimal depression
8 – 17	Mild
18 – 25	Moderate
26+	Severe

Fig. 2.1 Hamilton Depression Rating Scale (HAMD). (From Hamilton M 1960. Journal of Neurology, Neurosurgery and Psychiatry 23:56–62.)

Box 2.2   CORE SYMPTOMS OF DEPRESSION

- Sadness
- Loss of interest
- Poor appetite
- Sleep difficulty
- Loss of energy
- Pessimism or guilt
- Suicidal ideation

2.12

What are the physical symptoms of depression?

Poor sleep, especially frequent waking during the night and early morning waking, are of diagnostic importance in depression. Loss of appetite and weight loss of as much as 5% of body weight per month and constipation are other indicative biological features of depression. Tiredness and lethargy and general psychomotor retardation are also indicative, although sometimes the converse is true, and patients have an increase in appetite and put on weight and have hypersomnia. Thus, these physical symptoms are of considerable diagnostic interest, but not pathognomonic of depression.

Patients may exhibit retardation with poverty of facial expression, sparse and slow speech and a general slowing of thinking with difficulty in formulating ideas and an inability to make decisions. Other patients may be agitated with restlessness involving pacing, fidgeting and the same thought recurring constantly without any action being taken. Other features include a loss of libido or sexual drive with possible impotence or frigidity, muscle pains and difficulty coping with physical tasks at work.

2.13

When is treatment appropriate for patients who say they are depressed?

Depression should be treated when patients ask for help, when the illness is so severe as to cause significant disability, and when symptoms are persistent enough to warrant intervention. Ultimately, patients should be offered treatment if treatment is likely to help. If symptoms have been present for a few weeks, they are worthy of treatment.

2.14

Are people who never seem to feel happy depressed?

The answer depends on making the distinction between unhappiness and depression. The difference is primarily a qualitative one depending upon the severity of the symptoms, their chronicity and the degree of functional impairment. It is also a question of state and trait. Trait is a long-term personality factor which tends to remain relatively constant throughout life. States vary according to situations and internal and external variations. Some people are born pessimists who carry the world's burdens on their shoulders. They may be regarded as having a depressive personality or dysthymia.

2.15

What predisposes people to depressive illness?

Some people react better to adverse situations and therefore do not succumb to depression very easily, while others do not seem to have the emotional wherewithal to cope and they become depressed easily. The key to this lies in individual variability and nature and nurture. Vulnerability factors include a genetic predisposition. Other biological variables suggest that people are susceptible to developing depression at certain periods in their lives and not at others, providing an adequate stimulus arises. Psychological predeterminants would affect the individual's learned ability to react to stress. People who have learned to be more self-assured and to cope with stress are less likely to develop depression when challenged than those who have learned to cope poorly. There is also the question of the nature of the adverse situation. For example the loss of a parent may have a major impact on someone who continues to live in the family home and have much less impact if that person has not seen that parent for 20 years.

The contributing or trigger factors are discussed in Chapter 4.

2.16

How can we improve our performance in the diagnosis of depression?

The most important thing is to have a high index of suspicion for diagnosing depression since it is a common condition. Depression should always be considered in patients with non-specific somatic symptoms and those with a 'fat file'. Elderly patients with recent memory loss may not be dementing but have depressive illnesses. Another common feature of depressive illness is the recent onset of self-medication with alcohol. Many patients suffer from more than one condition: depressive disorders may be present but go unnoticed in people who have other physical, or even psychiatric, disturbances.

Screening questionnaires for patients and checklists for doctors are also helpful (Fig. 2.2).

Things to think about with a depressed patient

Name		Date	Date	Date
Ask about				
Physical complaints including pain				
Fatigue/insomnia				
Loss of concentration				
Difficulty in making decisions				
Loss of interest or pleasure				
Low mood or sadness				
Abnormal self-reproach, pessimism				
Inability to feel				
Weeping, shame				
Loss of interest in normal pleasures				
Unable to cope				
Feeling hopeless/helpless				
Wish to escape				
Ideas of self harm or suicide				
Warning signs				
Substantial suicide risk				
Excitement, rapid speech, history of mania				
Heavy alcohol use				
Drug treatment				
Drug and dosage				
Side effects				
Drug change				
Date drug started				
Date drug stopped				
Other options				
Counselling				
Relaxation or cognitive therapy				
Community psychiatric nurse				
Social worker				
Referral to psychiatrist				

Fig. 2.2 Depression patient checklist for doctors. (Adapted checklist from Glenwood Health Centre, Glenrothes, Fife.)

3 MANIFESTATIONS OF ANXIETY AND DEPRESSION

Introduction

Careful description of clinical syndromes, their definition and boundaries is of fundamental importance in research and in helping us define what we see and treat.

In the absence of clear biological markers for anxiety and depression, clinicians are basically dealing with abstract conditions diagnosed on symptoms, and the basic diagnostic assumptions will heavily influence the final diagnostic classification. It depends upon how the syndromes are defined to start with.

3.1

How valid is the distinction between anxiety and depression?

Strong support for a distinction between depression and anxiety comes from work done in Newcastle, UK, which was primarily conducted on inpatients at the more severe end of the spectrum. This approach had the benefit of promoting more sophisticated research in the area, but has not really added a great deal to the understanding of the basic processes. More recent work has shown that the stability of the diagnoses over time is not so good. Many patients can be diagnosed as one on one occasion and the other later. If anything, the diagnosis of depression is more stable than that of anxiety. Many patients fulfil criteria for both conditions at the same time. For example, in about a third of cases of major depression and anxiety there is an overlap and two-thirds of cases overlap when comparing minor depression and anxiety disorders. In patients diagnosed with anxiety disorders, about half would overlap with depression. Similarly, two-thirds of patients with agoraphobia and panic could also be diagnosed as having major depression.

3.2

Is it important to differentiate between anxiety and depression when treating patients?

Depression used to be treated with antidepressants, while benzodiazepines and counselling were given to patients with anxiety disorders. This distinction no longer holds true since the use of benzodiazepines for longer than a brief course of treatment is now discouraged. The two conditions have considerable overlap in their clinical features (see Question 3.3), and patients who present with depression at one time may well later present with anxiety symptoms and vice versa. Counselling and cognitive techniques are probably effective in both conditions, and antidepressants are also effective. MAOIs are particularly effective in anxiety/depressive states. Buspirone is the one exception, which appears to be more effective in anxiety than depression at normal therapeutic doses. The current view would be to treat the most prominent symptoms by the most appropriate means.

Since most treatments are effective for either condition and most patients seen in general practice have a mixed picture, the new diagnostic category of mixed anxiety and depression in the ICD10 should be welcome (see Table 1.1). The debate, however, will continue to reign. It is often most useful simply to ask patients whether they are more depressed than anxious or vice versa.

From a prognostic point of view it appears that depression has a better outcome than anxiety in its more severe forms. It would appear that panic disorder may be a separate clinical entity, although the same therapeutic principles apply. In most cases in general practice the distinction between anxiety and depression is not very helpful, although it may have some validity in the more serious cases referred to psychiatrists.

3.3

What are the similarities and differences between anxiety and depression?

The rating scales for anxiety and depression have many symptoms in common, such as sleep disturbance, anxiety, agitation, gastrointestinal disturbance and general somatic symptoms. Hypochondriasis is also present in both, as are intellectual and sexual problems. Key symptoms of depression are sadness, depressed mood, guilt and suicidal ideation with psychomotor retardation and general inability to enjoy pleasure. Features of high validity in diagnosing anxiety include fears, panic attacks, blushing, marked agoraphobia, derealization, and an age of onset under 35.

Box 3.1   SYMPTOMS WHICH DISCRIMINATE BETWEEN DEPRESSION AND ANXIETY

Anxiety
- Fears
- Panic attacks
- Blushing
- Marked agoraphobia
- Derealization

Depression
- Sadness
- Depressed mood
- Guilt
- Suicidal ideation
- Psychomotor retardation
- Loss of pleasure

33

Box 3.2 SYMPTOMS WHICH ARE COMMON TO ANXIETY AND DEPRESSION

- Tension
- Poor sleep
- Anxiety
- Agitation
- Somatic complaints

3.4

Is there any instrument that can be used to help discriminate between anxiety and depression?

A scale, which was devised by Zigmond and Snaith, and is simple and quick to use for distinguishing between anxiety and depression. A score of 7 or less is non-case, 8 to 10 a doubtful case, and 11 or more a definite case, for both depression and anxiety (see Fig. 1.1).

3.5

Is anxiety less serious than depression?

This of course depends on how the severity of the illness and 'seriousness' are quantified. Depression tends to be a more benign illness with exacerbations and remissions. In its more severe form it is associated with a significant mortality through suicide, and, although there are repeated exacerbations, there are often prolonged remissions during which the patient functions entirely normally. Anxiety on the other hand is often a milder illness, but in its chronic form can be extremely disabling. In any practice there must be more patients severely incapacitated by anxiety than by, for example, an illness known to cause chronic disability such as schizophrenia. Anxiety generally pursues a more chronic course, and although probably 70% of patients with anxiety disorders are generally well within a year, there remain 30% of patients with this common condition who have severe residual disabilities.

3.6

Why are anxious patients more difficult to manage than depressed patients?

Anxious patients tend to doubt everything they are told and are terrified of change. They importune their doctor but do not seem to accept what is offered. This is part of their psychopathology. Again, they project their anxiety and worry onto their doctor, which draws the doctor into a situation that makes him or her less effective. They turn off therapeutic positivism and patients are aware of this. Depressed patients are generally more accepting and comply better with treatment.

ANXIETY DISORDERS

3.7

At what age do anxiety disorders usually present?

Anxiety disorders often develop on top of generally anxious personalities and these can be traced back to early childhood. This long-term personality characteristic is known as the anxiety trait. On top of this, people develop anxiety states which are variable.

Anxiety disorders tend to become manifest around the time of late adolescence and the early 20s and are rarely new illnesses after the age of 35. Conditions that are present or appear then are usually carried on from conditions that have developed earlier in life. Anxiety disorders presenting later in life should be regarded with suspicion since they may well be manifestations of other conditions, such as depression or organic states.

3.8

Do secondary problems arise from long-standing anxiety disorders?

Anxiety disorders can act as triggers to further problems. These can be grouped according to problems of the natural history of anxiety disorders. For example the relationship between depression and anxiety remains unclear. Many people who have anxiety disorders will develop depression in later life, and other neurotic disorders such as sleep disturbance, alcoholism and drug abuse. Another form of secondary characteristic of anxiety includes physical problems that develop as a result of long-standing somatic symptoms. Chronic clenching of the masseter muscles can result in arthritis of the temporomandibular joint, giving rise to chronic headaches, and bruxism (grinding of the teeth) can result in dental problems. Chronic stress and worry may result in duodenal ulcers and irritable bowel syndrome (IBS) which may persist when the underlying stresses are relieved. Chronic muscular tension can result in muscle aches, backache and other somatic symptoms. Psychologically, patients become hypochondriacal and preoccupied with illness. They may develop a dependency on their families and the medical services, requiring constant reassurance. They may develop avoidant behaviour in order to sidestep situations which they feel increase their anxiety. Chronic anxiety inevitably alters family dynamics, which may lead to marital problems or problems at work and loss of employment due to absenteeism. The list of possible problems that untreated neurosis may generate is infinite and individual, often depending on the individual's Achilles' heel.

PHOBIAS

3.9

Do phobias generally develop de novo or from a previous generalized anxiety disorder? Where both types of anxiety co-exist, should they be treated separately?

Phobias are generally separate conditions from generalized anxiety disorders. Phobias for snakes, spiders and mice etc., classically develop between the ages of about 7 and 12 as a result of some imprinting phenomenon when the individual has a susceptibility to develop a phobia. They generally remain specific, and the individual does not generalize to other types of anxiety or phobia. Anxiety symptoms only occur in the presence of or thinking about the phobic object. More generalized phobias, such as agoraphobia and claustrophobia, are usually the result of a panic attack occurring in some particular situation. The patient will do everything possible to avoid having another attack, which is attributed to the situation, and will go on to develop avoidant behaviour such as not going outdoors or into confined spaces. Similarly, social phobias often develop in a particular social situation where an unpleasant event, usually a physical experience of choking or an embarrassing incident, becomes generalized and the patient becomes frightened of encountering that situation again. Social phobias often develop in late adolescence and the early 20s.

3.10

What is the incidence of agoraphobia?

About 5% of people develop agoraphobia at some time during their life, and of these about 3% have it during any 6-month period. It is thus a relatively common condition which, once developed, tends to persist. It is notably about three times as common in women as men. Agoraphobia is characterized by marked fear and associated avoidance of being alone in public places from which escape might be difficult or where help might not be available. It is associated with a fear of sudden incapacitation and the fear of fainting or the need to go to the toilet. It is also associated with situations where escape is difficult, such as in crowds, tunnels or lifts, and thus a patient may suffer from agoraphobia and claustrophobia together.

The condition can be quite mild, from a general sense of discomfort experienced in a lift, for example, to a major disability resulting in a chronic incapacity, in which the patient may be unable to answer the front door unaccompanied and requires an escort to go out. It is often easier to go out in the dark than during the day.

Most agoraphobia can be traced back to a panic attack or similar unpleasant experience and an associated avoidance of situations which are regarded as triggering events. Patients are frightened to venture out on their own in case another attack occurs and they have no means of escape. About one in five cases of agoraphobia do not appear to be associated with panic attacks, and their causation is less clear. They are probably associated with a general anxiety about being away from the security of the home. Agoraphobic patients are often relatively calm and content when at home and only become anxious when required to leave the security of their environment. The condition is variable, with some days better than others.

37

Since most agoraphobic sufferers are married women the condition has been dubbed the 'housebound housewife syndrome'. Presumably, women who do not have the support of a husband are forced to combat their fears at an earlier stage and do not have the opportunity to develop the complex of dependent relationships and avoidance behaviour that results in the full-blown syndrome.

3.11

What is the treatment for phobias?

The classical treatment for phobias is systematic desensitization involving a gradual exposure to the feared object, where the patient learns to deal with the anxiety symptoms that result. The advantage of this approach is that it rapidly generalizes to produce an improvement of anxiety symptoms overall. For example, with a fear of flying, the patient may be encouraged to draw up a hierarchy of fears, first to look at pictures of aeroplanes, then to spend a day sitting in a café at an airport, before spending a day watching aeroplanes take off and land, then finding a model of an aeroplane at a museum or air display to sit inside before going on a short flight with a therapist. At each stage of the process the patient would be encouraged to learn how to relax, to think in a positive manner about his or her problems, and to be reassured of the safety procedures. The patient should not progress on to the next step before having mastered the previous step. This graduated approach usually works.

When generalized anxiety and phobic disorders co-exist, treatment of one often benefits the other. The danger of simply treating the anxiety symptoms in someone with a phobia is that the anxiety symptoms may reduce but the phobic avoidance may remain unchanged. This is a particular danger with the benzodiazepines and patients need to be told that, as anxiety levels reduce, they must face their feared objects for treatment to achieve any real benefits.

3.12

What distinguishes phobias from panic attacks?

Phobias are anxiety states induced by specific situations, such as open spaces, heights, spiders or snakes. The sufferer characteristically realizes his or her fears are unreasonable or excessive, and does not generally have symptoms in the absence of the feared object, which is usually avoided.

Panic attacks are episodes of intense dread often associated with bodily symptoms such as palpitations and tightness in the chest, with a fear of impending death. Most people suffer from a panic attack at some point in their lives, but severe attacks are remembered with an exquisite clarity. Patients suffering from panic disorder will remember the exact time and place of their first attack and will go to great lengths to avoid further ones.

There is of course considerable overlap between all of these anxiety disorders in clinical practice.

PANIC DISORDER

3.13

What is panic disorder?

Panic disorder is a newly emerging concept. About 3% of the population suffers from it in any 6-month period. It is characterized by sudden unexpected attacks of panic which are associated with intense fear, often of dying, and a range of physical symptoms such as palpitations, choking, dizziness, trembling and sweating. Often symptoms begin for no obvious reason and the patient develops 'catastrophic thinking' and feels he or she may be dying or going crazy. The panic subsides after minutes or an hour or so, but recurs with little or no warning within a few days. Attacks then occur, often with increasing frequency. This leads to avoidance of the situations in which the attack was previously experienced. This secondary avoidance may restrict the patient's lifestyle significantly. Some patients, although they experience few attacks, have a persistent fear of a further attack and continue avoidance.

Most patients with panic disorder report a decrease in work quality; two-thirds have either lost their job or taken reduced income, and half complain of an inability to drive. Thus it is a condition of considerable morbidity.

3.14

Is panic disorder a manifestation of anxiety or depression?

Only between one-quarter and one-eighth of patients with anxiety disorders have panic attacks as part of their syndrome. This raises the question whether panic disorder is distinct from anxiety disorders and from depressive illnesses. In general, the clinical features and natural history of the conditions do differ. The current view is that panic disorder is clinically distinct from generalized anxiety disorder, although there is considerable overlap.

3.15

Is panic disorder a separate psychological entity?

Whether panic disorder is part of a separate syndrome, or part of the anxiety / depressive spectrum remains controversial, although it is obviously a recognizable clinical syndrome. There is considerable overlap between generalized anxiety symptoms and panic disorder, and a half to three-quarters of panic patients also have depressive illnesses at some stage. Approximately one-third of patients with depression also have panic attacks.

3.16

What causes panic attacks?

Panic attacks often come on 'out of the blue', in predisposed individuals who are under some mild stress. They often occur in previously healthy and anxiety-free individuals. A dramatic example was a shipwright who was playing poker with his friends. He picked up four aces and the excitement of the moment triggered his first panic attack. Over the next weeks he experienced further attacks and developed a chronic and disabling illness.

Panic attacks develop as a result of the misinterpretation of some relatively innocuous stimulus, such as dizziness, palpitations or a hot flush. Patients with panic disorder often have a mitral valve prolapse which can cause a benign cardiac arrhythmia. Others appear to hyperventilate, altering the acid–base balance of the blood and resulting in symptoms of light-headedness which may be misinterpreted as having a stroke. On the biological front, treating patients with lactic acid infusions which alter the pH of the blood can often precipitate panic attacks, as can giving patients drugs which have an opposite effect to benzodiazepines at the benzodiazepine receptor. Thus, panic attacks may have a physiological basis with a strong cognitive overlay.

3.17
What are the factors that precipitate panic attacks?

When considering the causation of panic attacks, it is necessary to distinguish between the mechanisms and the effects. The mechanisms are complex and ill-understood, but involve a genetic predisposition and various physical triggers, such as palpitations. Some patients find cues, for example dizziness or hyperventilation with finger tingling, as the unpleasant stimulus. Patients then develop catastrophic thinking around the event and interpret this relatively minor stimulus as a symptom of a major problem with impending doom. A vicious circle of fear and escalating symptoms arises and a full-blown panic attack occurs.

Once patients have been so distressed by an attack, they avoid situations and cues which they believe will precipitate another attack. Thus avoidance behaviour develops for potential triggering situations. Patients become so frightened of having a further attack that they develop a 'fear of the fear'.

Though the original stimulus, often a simple physiological event, may be unknown, patients become preoccupied with psychological cues or events which may trigger these sometimes spontaneous events.

3.18
What is the best treatment for panic disorder?

The best treatment is early diagnosis and strong reassurance and explanation of the event so that the patient does not develop into a chronic neurotic after a couple of attacks. Since it is likely that attacks will recur, patients should be reassured that they are not harmful, and

41

are a relatively normal phenomenon. Most people will experience at least one attack during their lifetime, and they should be encouraged to regard these as harmless and normal.

Once the attacks are established and recurrent, treatment options are more complex. Psychological treatments involving relaxation and anxiety management are favoured by many. Patients learn the mechanisms of attacks and how to reassure themselves that they are dealing with a normal phenomenon which will pass. They should learn to alter thinking, switch thoughts and develop relaxation techniques to abort attacks, or prevent them escalating.

The alternative is to use medication. Benzodiazepines may be prescribed acutely for occasional short-term use and beta-blockers may prove helpful for cardiac symptoms. Antidepressants are generally effective in blocking attacks, even if they occur in the absence of depressive symptoms. Traditionally, imipramine has been the drug of choice, given at a starting dose of 10 mg for a few days, and increasing gradually over a matter of a couple of weeks to a dose of 150 mg per 24-hour period (possibly given as a once-nightly dose). Some patients may have their attacks controlled with much lower doses. The problem with this treatment is that it is associated with the various antidepressant side effects, and that, unless the medication is increased very gradually, it may well aggravate attacks initially. Thus patients who are already developing phobias arising from situations that may precipitate anxiety will become phobic of medication. The newer SSRIs are also effective in blocking panic attacks and have a better side-effect profile, although they can also worsen panic attacks initially. MAOIs are effective in panic disorder but, again, need to be taken for a matter of some weeks to be truly effective. Their side-effect profile is generally more favourable in panic sufferers, and they are probably the pharmacological treatment of choice, but they are associated with serious and potentially fatal side effects if combined with tyramine-containing foods, and are therefore not the treatment of first choice. It remains to be seen how effective the new reversible monoamine oxidase inhibitors (RIMAs) are. High doses of benzodiazepines, especially alprazolam, will block panic attacks, but the dangers of habituation are substantial and patients have real difficulty stopping them. Although they work more quickly, their long-term use is not recommended. With pharmacological treatments, symptoms may recur when treatment is stopped.

When treating patients with panic disorder, it is important not only to block the number of attacks, but also to reduce avoidance behaviour.

Patients have to be encouraged to overcome their phobias, not just to reduce the number of attacks.

Treatment of the acute episode is ideally by reassurance, although in extreme cases a short course of benzodiazepines could be administered. Rebreathing from a paper bag probably has more of a placebo effect rather than a physiological one.

Ultimately, the treatment of choice depends upon what patients are prepared to accept or want. Psychological treatments have a lot to recommend them, at least as a first line of treatment. If reassurance and explanation fail, then antidepressant medication should be considered. It may need to be continued for some time, since panic can become a chronic disorder.

INSOMNIA

3.19

Does insomnia exist as an independent condition or is it always secondary to some other factor such as depression, anxiety, hunger, etc.?

Insomnia is an extremely common presenting problem in general practice. Patients frequently complain that either they cannot fall asleep easily, or cannot stay asleep for a sufficiently long time. Primary insomnia exists in about half of the sufferers in whom poor sleep is constitutional. In the other half, insomnia is a symptom of an underlying disease process, often psychiatric or emotional disturbance (Table 3.1).

Table 3.1   Common sleep disturbance syndromes and their first-line treatment

Syndrome	Treatment
Disrupted sleep pattern, constitutionally light sleep	Sleep habit training
Acute insomnia, jet lag	Short-acting hypnotic (2 or 3 nights)
Chronic insomnia	Sleep habit training Intermittent hypnotics Exclude depression

Table 3.1   Common sleep disturbance syndromes and their first-line treatment *Cont'd*

Syndrome	Treatment
Depression	Antidepressants
Reduced sleep in elderly	Sleep habit training Avoid hypnotics Short-acting ones only
Physical illness	Treat primary condition Analgesia Hypnotics if appropriate
Alcoholism/drug abuse	No hypnotics
Children	Behavioural programmes Habit training Support parents
Sleep apnoea	Sleep specialist, ear nose and throat (ENT) surgeon, chest physician
Hypnotic dependency	Gradual withdrawal, if appropriate

3.20

What proportion of the population suffers from true insomnia?

About 50% of people admit to poor sleep at some time; about 30% report sleep difficulties in any one year, and about 15% of patients have what might be regarded as insomnia. 11 million prescriptions for sleeping pills are written annually in the UK, mostly for elderly long-term users.

Insomnia is a complex issue which has many components. There is the duration of sleep, the quality of sleep, and the subjective feeling of its quality and whether one wakes refreshed or tired in the morning. Many patients complain of very bad sleep but actually when observed sleep quite normally during the night (Fig. 3.1).

A sleep questionnaire

• *How long did it take you to fall asleep after going to bed?*

☐ 5 min ☐ 10 min ☐ 15 min

☐ 20 min ☐ 30 min ☐ 45 min

☐ 1 hour ☐ more than 1 hour

• *Compared to the time it normally takes you to fall asleep, was it*

☐ very much quicker ☐ much quicker ☐ quicker

☐ as normal ☐ slower ☐ much slower

☐ very much slower

• *Compared to normal, did you sleep*

☐ longer than usual ☐ as usual ☐ less than usual

• *Did you sleep*

☐ more deeply than usual ☐ as usual ☐ more lightly than usual

• *How did you feel on waking up?*

☐ much more alert ☐ more alert ☐ alert

☐ as usual ☐ drowsy ☐ more drowsy

☐ much more drowsy

Fig. 3.1 Patient questionnaire for insomnia.

3.21

Should I prescribe hypnotics for insomnia?

The first issue is to make a diagnosis of the nature of the problem. Initial insomnia may arise from anxiety, early morning waking from a depressive illness, reduced sleep time because of ageing, poor subjective sleep because of too much alcohol in the evening, or the myriad other reasons for the subjective complaint of insomnia. By taking a broad history, the problem becomes clearer and the solution apparent. Relief of pain, reassurance, support and the treatment of depressive illnesses are important. You could consider alternatives to sleeping pills such as self-help material and audio cassettes, and you could offer general advice on sleep hygiene.

You may consider a short course of hypnotics appropriate – in this case a week's supply of sleeping pills, to be taken as required and not every night, in order to help the patient over a short-term crisis. The patient should understand that sleeping tablets are not a long-term solution, and will not be prescribed in the long term.

3.22
What are the qualities to look for in a hypnotic drug?

The ideal hypnotic should rapidly, pleasantly and reliably induce sleep. It should be as normal a sleep as possible without disturbing the normal physiology of sleep patterns. It should allow the patient to awake refreshed without hangover. It should be effective from the first night, and its effects should last for several nights without rebound insomnia when it is discontinued.

3.23
Which drugs best approach this ideal profile?

A drug which is relatively rapidly absorbed, and has a duration of action of approximately 6 hours. This would correspond to a relatively short half-life compound. It should certainly have a half-life of less than 24 hours since, if it were longer, the drug would accumulate. There is, as always, considerable inter-individual variation in the pharmacokinetics of these drugs; their duration of action can vary enormously. Triazolam was a good drug, although its duration of action was rather short in some people, and, because of its potency and rapid elimination, some people developed adverse effects and it was withdrawn (see page 104, 6.6). Zopiclone, zolpidem, chlormethiazole, lormetazepam, temazepam and loprazolam have appropriate pharmacokinetic profiles, although chlormethiazole can cause nasal stuffiness, zopiclone gives a bad taste and temazepam is prone to abuse by drug addicts. Chloral hydrate is another good drug, but dangerous in overdose. Nitrazepam and flurazepam are not appropriate because of the long half-lives of their metabolites in chronic use.

3.24

What precautions should I take when prescribing hypnotic drugs?

You should be sure you are not missing a treatable depressive illness, for which antidepressants should be prescribed, or any other treatable primary pathology. Patients should be warned about the risk of dependence and should not be offered repeat prescriptions or issued more than a week's supply of medication at a time. Ideally the prescription should not be repeated unless there are exceptional circumstances. The patient should take them every second or third night and be warned that hypnotics are not a long-term solution.

3.25

There are now several hypnotics available over the counter, some of which contain powerful antihistamines. Do you think this is a good idea?

For years we have been trying to get away from antihistamines as sedatives because of the slow onset of action and also their long half-lives resulting in hangover effects. If patients really need medication they would be better off taking one of the more modern sleeping pills such as zopiclone or zolpidem which are tried and tested. The danger is that patients may use self-medication for insomnia which is a symptom of a treatable depression. On the other hand taking an occasional over-the-counter hypnotic is probably not all that harmful.

3.26

Should patients who have taken barbiturates over a long time continue to take them?

In many practices there will be a few patients who have been prescribed barbiturates for night sedation for many years.

It is worth trying to switch them over to benzodiazepines at least. Patients' tolerance may decrease with age and confusion and chronic intoxication may develop. Having said this, if patients are unable to

47

switch or discontinue them and are stabilized on them, it is appropriate to prescribe these drugs as necessary while monitoring the situation.

3.27

What advice do you have for a patient who is worried about sleeping problems?

Having excluded a treatable depressive illness, I would give advice on general sleep habit training (see Box 3.3) which includes regular bedtime, moderate exercise, avoiding caffeine and alcohol, and the practice of relaxation and thought-stopping techniques which can be learned from self-help tapes or books.

Box 3.3   SLEEP HABIT TRAINING

- Self-monitoring
- Regular bedtime and rising
- Sleep only as much as is needed
- No daytime naps
- Regular exercise
- No alcohol or caffeine late in the day
- If you cannot sleep, do not lie in bed and brood – get up and do something
- Practise progressive muscular relaxation
- Avoid excessive noise and heat in the bedroom
- Occasional sleeping pills are OK

HYPOCHONDRIASIS

3.28

What is hypochondriasis?

Hypochondriasis is the preoccupation with the belief or fear of having a serious disease. It is based on the misinterpretation of physical signs and sensations which hypochondriacs ascribe to physical illness. The belief is held despite proper examination and investigation of the complaint and persists despite medical reassurance. Some patients are misinterpreting the somatic features of anxiety and panic disorder, and in rare instances patients have somatic delusions. It is often found as part of a depressive syndrome, or in patients with severe anxiety, but is more common in people with abnormal personalities and an introspective disposition. Like so many conditions, it varies in intensity.

There are many variations on hypochondriasis. Patients may have cardiac neurosis or a preoccupation with abdominal complaints (hence hypo-chondrium). They often have some measure of physical disorder, but their fear of the disorder is quite out of proportion to its severity. Hypochondria is generally regarded as secondary to an underlying psychiatric process.

3.29

How does hypochondria differ from anxiety disorder with prominent physical symptoms?

Hypochondria differs from the somatic symptoms of anxiety in the degree of the preoccupation with the fear of the disease, rather than the symptom itself. Many patients with hypochondria have developed it on top of panic attacks or other somatic features of anxiety and the hypochondria is an elaboration of the somatic anxiety.

It should not be confused with malingering, where a patient consciously presents features of an illness in order to achieve a goal, or with hysteria, where a patient subconsciously develops symptoms or alterations in physical functioning suggesting a physical disorder because of psychological stresses. Hysteria is a very rare condition. Another common variant is somatization disorder where patients have many physical symptoms or are preoccupied with their ill-health, and have many different symptoms in various bodily systems without obvious organic causation. This condition often starts in early adulthood and persists for many years. Mild forms of hypochondria probably relate to a generally anxious predisposition and anxious personality, and many hypochondriacal complaints are actually somatic manifestations of anxiety.

3.30

In hypochondria, is there an element of depression as well as anxiety about health?

In cases where patients are severely depressed, they are deluded that they have a grave internal disorder, for example their bowels are clogged up and they are empty inside. Hypochondriacal preoccupation is also a common feature of less severe forms of depression, and is more commonly seen in cultures in which depression is somatized. Patients may even develop hysterical conversion symptoms in a manner that was observed in Vienna at the end of the 19th century. In these hypochondriacal forms of depression, anxiety about the presumed physical disorder is notably absent.

3.31

How should I treat hypochondriasis?

You should exclude, or treat, any obvious underlying pathology, such as depression or anxiety. If in doubt, a course of antidepressants is indicated. A cognitive approach is often helpful. Patients are asked to interpret the significance of their symptoms and explore all the possibilities, ranging from terminal cancer to normal bodily function as potential causes, ranking them in order of likelihood. The likelihood of each possibility should be discussed. Patients should be encouraged to repeat this process every time they develop their fears or symptoms. A low dose of an antipsychotic agent, such as pimozide or sulpiride, may be indicated if the patient is deluded. If hysteria is suspected, the patient should be referred to a competent physician to exclude organic pathology, since hysteria is a very rare condition these days, and usually a misdiagnosed genuine pathology.

Treatment is directed at the underlying condition, with antidepressants or appropriate anxiolytics, together with reassurance, explanation and appropriate investigation. It is important not to over-investigate hypochondriacal patients. In some instances, a psychodynamic explanation of the meaning of the symptom and the fears associated with the unrealistic expectation of illness is justified. For example, headaches can be interpreted as symptomatic of a brain tumour, if a close friend died of a brain tumour. It is important to know what level of investigation a patient would find acceptable, and for the treating doctor to decide what level of referral and investigation is appropriate.

In the most severe form of depression, ECT may be the treatment of choice (Ch. 7).

OBSESSIVE COMPULSIVE DISORDER (OCD)

3.32
What are the features of OCD?

OCD is characterized by persistent thoughts or impulses which are acknowledged by the patient to be irrational but which recur despite resistance. After some time, resistance tends to wane since the thoughts and resulting rituals continue to recur, and resistance is accompanied by an increase in anxiety. The obsessional thoughts and rituals are time-consuming and interfere with social relationships and jobs. The original thought is the obsession, which may result in a compulsion to perform a certain act. For example, if the obsessional thought is that the hands are dirty, the compulsion is usually to wash them. If this is not possible the patient becomes extremely anxious.

OCD is a chronic and fluctuating condition, but, unlike many conditions in the anxiety spectrum, it is highly stable and specific.

3.33
What is the aetiology of OCD?

The aetiology of OCD is uncertain, although drugs acting on 5-HT reuptake appear to have a specific action in this syndrome. Neurological involvement such as heavy metal poisoning and basal ganglia disease may also be related.

Recent research has found neuroanatomical abnormalities in the occipitofrontal cortex and caudate nucleus in patients suffering from OCD. Neuro-imaging studies using SPECT scanners which measure metabolic activity in vivo, have demonstrated changes in activity in the caudate nucleus when compared to normals. Unfortunately, the results are inconclusive, some studies showing increased activity and others decreased activity. It has been suggested that there may be hyperactive circuits in OCD between the orbitofrontal cortex and the caudate nucleus, which are linked by glutaminergic fibres. Unfortunately, this remains unproven. Biological markers of the disease remains enigmatic.

Clearly, psychological theories relating to its causation are important because the other mainstay of treatment has been behaviour therapy. Classical psychoanalysis has little to offer in this condition and is contraindicated.

3.34

Should OCD be considered part of the anxiety spectrum?

OCD is traditionally classified among anxiety disorders because resisting obsessions evokes anxiety. It is increasingly being seen as a disorder distinct from other psychiatric disorders by virtue of its unique and strange clinical syndrome with symptoms quite unlike any other condition. Obsessive thoughts appear to be central to the condition, and the anxiety secondary. The response to medication appears to be distinct from other conditions both in its time course and in the specificity of the medication. For example, SSRIs appear to have an anti-obsessional action, independent of whether the patient has significant anxiety or depressive symptoms or not. Depressive symptoms improve faster with SSRI medication than obsessive symptoms. Also, the behavioural treatments for OCD are aimed at confronting anxieties by resisting obsessions and then learning to reduce anxiety, rather than by dealing with the primary obsession.

3.35

What is the most effective agent in the treatment of OCD?

The most extensively studied drug for the treatment of OCD is clomipramine, but amitriptyline is also effective, and the effects of these tricyclics appear to be independent of their antidepressant action. Fluvoxamine has also been shown to be effective and the other SSRIs would appear to be as effective. The response tends to be slow over many weeks, and an overall response rate is about 60% with residual obsessional symptoms remaining. Higher doses than used in the treatment of depression are needed. Thus, the pharmacological treatment of OCD is not dramatic, although useful benefits, with significant improvement in the patient's social functioning, are possible.

HYSTERIA

3.36

What is hysteria?

In hysteria, patients have a loss of or alteration to physical functioning which suggests a physical disorder, but which is thought to be caused or aggravated by psychological mechanisms. These are unconscious with the purpose of some gain. The classic example is of a woman who could not swallow water because she witnessed a dog drinking from her dying father's glass of water at his bedside. Drinking water, which reminded her of her ambivalent feelings towards her father, resulted in anxiety. Patients with hysterical conversion symptoms are usually surprisingly devoid of anxiety symptoms ('la belle indifférence') because of their use of this defence mechanism. They develop hysterical symptoms because of an inability to cope with the anxiety of some situation or thoughts. They then develop the mental dynamism of converting anxieties into physical symptoms.

Hysteria is a rare condition in Britain. More commonly seen in emerging societies, it usually occurs as a secondary phenomenon to other psychiatric disorders, most notably depression. Hysteria tends to be a diagnosis of desperation when no other explanation can be found to account for a series of symptoms. At this point the doctor should reconsider the diagnosis.

Hysteria probably exists more commonly in a minor form where patients, for unconscious reasons, often associated with realistic anxiety, tend to exaggerate the disabilities associated with real physical illness. In such cases, support and reassurance are often helpful.

3.37

What is the treatment for hysteria?

True hysteria is a difficult condition to treat. There is no accepted way of dealing with it except that underlying conditions such as anxiety and depression or schizophrenia should be dealt with by medication or

53

counselling. Abreaction with pentothal often has dramatic, if temporary, effects. A behavioural approach is often indicated, and classically psychoanalysis is advocated, although the results are uncertain since patients rarely persist with treatment.

3.38

What are hysterical outbursts?

These are gross dissociative states often resulting from an acute situation or crisis, and often superimposed on hysterical personality disorders. Such people are prone to excessive emotionality and attention-seeking behaviour. They frequently seek and demand reassurance and have exaggerated emotional expressions with temper tantrums and uncontrollable sobbing, or excessive ardour, depending on the situation. They are often self-centred. As such, under relatively minor provocation they may have excessive emotional outbursts.

3.39

How should hysterical outbursts be treated?

The treatment for the acute episode is to provide comfort, reassurance and mild restraint if applicable. A gentle, non-confrontational approach of support and sympathy is best. Occasional one-off doses of anxiolytics may be indicated if the situation is seriously out of control. The treatment of the underlying hysterical personality disorder is more difficult, since these conditions are notoriously inaccessible to management. They develop in early adulthood, and tend to settle down slowly in the fourth decade of life. The management of these conditions is to deal with the crises until spontaneous improvement occurs in time.

DEPRESSIVE DISORDERS
Agitated depression

3.40
What is agitated depression?

Some depressed patients express their anxiety symptoms in physical activity or agitation. This can range from mild restlessness to ceaseless movement with hand-wringing or skin-picking. Pressure of speech is usually present and the individual talks incessantly about the same topics. Patients may importune and fasten on doctors and nurses demanding reassurance and help. Difficulty in concentration occurs and patients cannot focus on the task in hand. They cannot stop thinking about the unpleasant things they do not wish to think about. Agitation is more common, and more marked, in depression occurring in middle life or older age.

3.41
What is the best treatment for agitated depression?

Antidepressants should be used for the treatment of depressive symptoms. If patients are distressed and anxious as well, then it is appropriate to treat them with benzodiazepines for 2 or 3 weeks while the antidepressants begin to have an effect. Other alternatives are to prescribe a sedative antidepressant or a low-dose neuroleptic, but the important point is to give full doses of antidepressants.

Smiling depression

3.42
What is meant by smiling depression?

This is a term used to describe patients who present at interview with denial of a depressed mood and maintain a smiling exterior. The smile, however, lacks warmth and spontaneity. Referral for medical advice is usually at the instigation of a close relative or associate who has noticed a change in the patient's behaviour, such as a falling off of efficiency at work, slowing down in thought or movement or withdrawal from social contact. Psychiatrists are often particularly worried when they encounter such people who are otherwise very depressed. It may be that the patient has arrived at the decision to commit suicide and is now pretending to be cheerful in order to mask the depression and avoid suspicion while planning suicide.

Brief recurrent depression

3.43
What is brief recurrent depression?

This is an increasingly recognized condition where the patient has quite severe and disabling bouts of depression lasting about 3 days. The individual becomes tense, touchy and irritable as well as awkward in relationships with others, and is often misdiagnosed as having a personality disorder. Such a patient is at particular risk of suicidal behaviour during depressive phases. He or she suffers from a range of symptoms seen in major depression, but the illness has a sudden onset. The episodes terminate rather suddenly, but have a tendency to recur after a few weeks.

The sudden change from apparent normality to severe depression is difficult, not only for the individual but also for relatives and colleagues. The impulsiveness of sufferers often results in suicide attempts.

3.44
How should recurrent brief depression be treated?

Antidepressants are not particularly helpful because the patient will be in spontaneous remission of the brief episode before they take effect. There is also the risk that antidepressants may provide the means for attempting suicide by overdose during the next episode. They may have a slight prophylactic effect. Low-dose neuroleptics, such as 20 mg flupenthixol injections monthly, may reduce recurrent suicidal behaviour. Lithium or SSRIs may be of some use, as may MAOIs. Supportive psychotherapy is of potential value, but deep psychotherapy may increase the risk of suicide. The condition remains difficult to define and treat.

Dysthymia

3.45

What is dysthymia?

This is a low-grade grumbling depression with symptoms present most days for a couple of years. Patients must present with a depressed mood plus two other depressive symptoms. The symptoms are mild and chronic. Many of these patients will have major depression which has been partly or inadequately treated, and many patients have chronic dysthymia with episodic major depressions (double depression).

Seasonal affective disorder (SAD)

3.46

What is SAD?

Although the diagnosis is new, the concept was hypothesized by Hippocrates, and by other observers since then. The cardinal features are recurrent mood cycles with depression usually starting around October/November and lifting in March or April, when there is often a mild hypomanic swing. The mood abnormality is not particularly severe, although it is sufficient to cause distress to the sufferer and those around him or her.

3.47

What are the symptoms of SAD?

Irritability is a common symptom of SAD, as is weight change, either weight loss, but more commonly, significant weight gain during the winter which is lost during the summer. Sufferers experience work difficulties and problems with interpersonal relationships as well as problems with libido, concentration and energy and various physical symptoms such as aches and pains. In general, the symptoms of SAD are those of depression of moderate severity.

3.48
How can SAD be treated?

The specific treatment is artificial phototherapy with lights providing 2500 lux from full-spectrum lights for 4 hours a day. A treatment response should be noted within 4 or 5 days if it will occur, but treatment then has to be maintained throughout the winter months or the patient needs to move to a sunnier climate.

Bipolar disorder

3.49
What is bipolar disorder?

This condition is sometimes referred to as manic-depressive psychosis. Variations in mood from time to time are universally experienced as part of natural cyclothymia, but manic-depressive psychosis would imply a severity of the illness at the psychotic end of the spectrum and is therefore very serious. In this condition, patients are prone to recurrent episodes of depressive illness, but also episodes of mania, where they exhibit features of a heightened mood with cheerfulness, elation and euphoria. Irritability and hostility are also common, as is overactive behaviour. There is racing of thought with rapid speech and writing. Patients have flights of ideas and erratic changes of thoughts resulting in thought disorder with increasingly tenuous connections between the thoughts. Punning, clang associations and rhyming are common. Manic patients usually feel very well and have little insight into their difficulties. Although superficially a state of mania seems an attractive condition, it can be very destructive since patients can in a few days spend vast amounts of money, commit serious sexual indiscretions and do profound damage to themselves professionally and in their relationships. They are difficult to treat because of their lack of insight, and in elderly patients there is a risk of physical exhaustion because of overactivity.

3.50

Can both phases of bipolar mood disorder be present simultaneously?

Some patients exhibit both manic and depressive features at the same time, and this is called a mixed affective state.

3.51

How common is bipolar mood disorder?

Manic depression is much less common than depression by itself. Estimates vary, but major depression is about four times as common as bipolar depression.

3.52

Which drug should be used in the prophylaxis of bipolar disorder, and for how long?

Lithium prophylaxis is the drug of choice for the treatment of bipolar disorder. If this fails, carbamazepine, neuroleptics or sodium valproate may be second- and third-line treatments, either alone or in combination. For unipolar depressions, the choice lies between antidepressants and lithium. Both are probably equally effective, and considerations of side effects, cost and the need for monitoring of plasma concentrations are important in governing choice. These are long-term treatments. If, having embarked on therapy, the patient benefits from treatment, it is probably best to continue indefinitely with annual reviews. Again, the quality of remission on treatment has to be balanced against the side effects and risks of treatment and the condition of the patient prior to prophylaxis, before deciding whether to continue treatment after a period of years.

Prophylaxis is dealt with in more detail in Chapter 8.

4 CONTRIBUTING OR TRIGGER FACTORS

Introduction

Psychosocial factors have an impact on our ability to withstand and cope with stress and the development of anxiety and depression. Stressors also prevent people from recovering adequately. An interactive model for understanding the relative contributions of social, psychological and biological factors is developing.

4.1

Are the stresses of contemporary life any greater than those of any other time?

There is no evidence, basically because the concept of stress is a relatively modern one, and epidemiological work was not undertaken until quite recently.

The consumption of laudanum (tincture of opium) equivalent to 150 doses per head of population per year was documented in the late 19th century. This may be comparable to the use of benzodiazepines today, and may be safely assumed to have been largely self-medication for anxiety. Although life has become physically less arduous and imminent dangers of death from disease and natural disaster have become less, people have lost the fatalism associated with these problems. There are current pressures such as unemployment and housing difficulties, but in times of comparative affluence, people worry more about themselves and their self-actualization, and at times of privation they worry more about basic needs such as warmth, shelter and safety from imminent danger, for example, during the Second World War people complained less of neurosis. People are most aware of their anxieties in highly affluent societies such as the east and west coasts of the United States and the capitals of the industrialized world. As they become more affluent, they are encouraged to express their anxieties more. In these circumstances, people have the time and money to worry about themselves. There is also the availability of therapists ready and willing to help them deal with their problems.

4.2

What sort of social factors are relevant in anxiety and depression?

Social factors are important in generating and maintaining anxiety and depression. It is reasonable to feel depressed if you are elderly, lonely, bereaved and isolated, and to be anxious if you live on a housing estate where you are frightened by the presence of delinquent youths. Poor accommodation, unfriendly neighbours, physical illness, recent accidents, loss of confidence, together with financial difficulties, add up to the social mix which can result in unhappiness. Young women who are stuck in a high-rise block with several young children and limited social outlets are at risk of developing depression. Early loss of the mother is also a risk factor for depression, presumably because modelling for adulthood is impaired. Ultimately chronic or, more particularly, acute social adversity can result in psychological decompensation and resultant anxiety and depression. Acute life events have been shown to be triggers for depressive illnesses and several minor adverse events may be cumulative, when one alone was not enough.

4.3

What cultural factors contribute to anxiety?

Anxiety is hard to define, and its expression is culturally determined. Thus, the prevalence results from an interaction of a genetic predisposition, a culturally bound definition, and the expectations of the individuals within a society as well as from environmental and social stresses.

Some cultures appear to manifest anxiety more than others. Classically, the Mediterranean temperament is volatile and allows the expression of emotions more freely than, for example, the stiff upper-lipped English. People living in more stressed environments are more prone to develop anxiety-related symptoms, and, in western society, people are inclined to complain more of emotional problems than in other societies. In Japanese culture, for example, where it is not acceptable to talk about one's feelings, erythrophobia (a fear of blushing) is a common complaint.

4.4

Does depression present differently in people of other cultures?

Depression is to a great extent culturally determined, and therefore it is important to develop an understanding of the concepts of different cultures. Very broadly speaking, patients from newly emerging cultures show hysterical somatization syndromes in many ways similar to those described by Freud in Vienna at the turn of the century. As a broad generalization, these patients tend to somatize their problems, complaining of bodily pains rather than psychological

63

symptoms. As well as diffuse and ill-defined maladies, they often have a very sorrowful look, which should be the clue to diagnosis. Other patients just look very depressed and complain of sleep disturbance. North Americans often express their difficulties in terms of poor relationships with others, a reflection of the influence of psychotherapy in their psychiatric thinking. These remarks are gross generalizations but they serve to highlight the need to keep an open mind when dealing with patients from different cultural backgrounds. If there is any doubt, it may be useful to seek advice from family members, although in my experience their misconceptions are just as bad as my own.

4.5

Why do some patients get better sooner than others?

Patients of upper social classes who are well educated and who see their problems as emotional, those whose problems have had recent onset, and patients who have had few previous treatments generally have a better prognosis than the converse. In other words, patients who are successful in life tend to be more successful in recovery from disease.

4.6

What factors influence the prognosis of the illness?

If a patient has a preference for drug treatment and consults a doctor who is happy prescribing medication, the patient is more likely to have a satisfactory outcome than if the patient wants medication and the doctor wants to offer counselling, or vice versa. Depressed patients generally have a better prognosis than those with anxiety. The doctor's attitude appears to be more important in the treatment of anxiety than depression. Men generally have a better prognosis than women. The more time a doctor spends with a patient, the better the prognosis, and patients seen in general practice generally do better than those referred to specialists since they are presumably the easier cases.

Patients who are well supported by family and social environment will have a better prognosis than those who are not, and this is particularly relevant to those with 'reactive-type' depression. Relatively straightforward depressive illnesses respond better than complex ones. Clearly the treatment used will be important. ECT is the most effective treatment for depression, and inadequate doses of antidepressants are rarely more effective than placebo. Medication is probably the most effective treatment for symptom relief, and psychological therapies have more to offer in terms of socialization and coming to terms with the effects of the illness. Of the greatest importance is the history of previous episodes and patients' response to therapy. The likelihood of recovery in people who have always been depressed is less than in those who have a short-lived illness. Depressive illnesses are easier to treat at a time when they would be undergoing natural resolution, and are harder to treat when they are still developing. Panic disorder is probably better treated early before secondary disabilities have had a chance to develop. Ultimately, the past is the best predictor to the future, and those patients who have had difficulties in previous illnesses will have a worse prognosis than those who have had minimal problems in the past.

STRESS

4.7

What are the effects of too much stress?

Stress is a non-specific stimulus which can unleash diseases at many specific sites, and affects individuals in different ways – we all have our individual Achilles' heel. Too much stress can affect mental and physical well-being, as well as giving rise to symptoms of anxiety and depression. It can act as a trigger for other major medical or psychiatric events, precipitating full-blown depressive or psychotic episodes, myocardial infarction or alcoholism in susceptible individuals. These disease processes may then continue of their own accord. Chronic stress also gives rise to peptic ulceration and hypertension and can aggravate diabetes and musculoskeletal problems.

4.8

What is the difference between stress and anxiety?

The two terms have considerable overlap and are often used incorrectly. Stress is the force exerted upon an individual. Environmental stressors and life events, such as family pressures and changes in work, can produce a feeling of being stressed. This is generally regarded as a normal response – some level of stress is desirable – but it can become excessive from time to time. Anxiety is a feeling, resulting from an interaction of external stressors, internal biological predispositions and psychological preparedness. In general, anxiety is regarded as pathological and undesirable.

4.9

How can stress be measured? Are there any reliable stress measuring scales which we can use?

Stress can be quantified by means of the rating scale of Holmes and Rahe. This is a reliable instrument which assesses stress over the past 12 months (Fig. 4.1).

4.10

What is the relationship between stress and performance?

The Yerkes Dodson Law shows that as arousal increases, so does performance. For example, while sitting relaxed, the level of performance is low as is the level of arousal. A stimulus, such as the doorbell ringing, increases arousal and a stressful situation provokes greater activity. Within normal situations, performance increases with increasing arousal. Beyond a certain level, however, arousal and associated anxiety can become counter-productive, resulting in impaired performance. For example, exam nerves or stage fright can result in people performing less well than expected. At a certain point they begin to decompensate.

Score patient's stress with Holmes and Rahe scale				
Event	**Score**			
Death of spouse	100 ☐	Son or daughter leaving home	29 ☐
Divorce	73 ☐	Trouble with in-laws	29 ☐
Marital separation	65 ☐	Outstanding personal achievement	28 ☐
Jail term	63 ☐	Spouse begins or stops work	26 ☐
Death of a close family member	63 ☐	Starting or finishing school	26 ☐
Personal injury or illness	53 ☐	Change in living conditions	25 ☐
Marriage	50 ☐	Change of personal habits	24 ☐
Loss of job	47 ☐	Trouble with boss	23 ☐
Marital reconciliation	45 ☐	Change in work hours or conditions	20 ☐
Retirement	45 ☐	Change in residence	20 ☐
Change in family member's health	44 ☐	Change in school	20 ☐
Pregnancy	40 ☐	Change in recreational habits	19 ☐
Sex difficulties	39 ☐	Change in church activities	19 ☐
Addition to family	39 ☐	Change in social activities	18 ☐
Business re-adjustment	39 ☐	Taking out a small mortgage/loan	17 ☐
Change in financial state	38 ☐	Change in sleeping habits	16 ☐
Death of a close friend	37 ☐	More/fewer family gatherings	15 ☐
Change to different type of work	36 ☐	Change in eating habits	15 ☐
More/less marital arguments	35 ☐	Holiday	13 ☐
Taking out a large mortgage or loan	31 ☐	Christmas	12 ☐
Foreclosure on mortgage or loan	30 ☐	Minor violation of the law	11 ☐
Change in work responsibilities	29 ☐	Total	

Assess your patient's stress score

Less than 150:	30% probability of developing an illness (no more than average risk)
Between 150 and 299:	50% probability of developing an illness
Over 300:	80% probability of developing an illness

Fig. 4.1   The Holmes and Rahe stress rating scale. (From Holmes I, Rahe R 1967. The social re-adjustment rating scale. Journal of Psychosomatic Research 11:213–218.)

Where individuals stand at a given moment on the performance curve, depends on their innate physiological and emotional reactivity, whether they are basically highly aroused or not, and on the severity of the arousing stimulus. Highly anxious people tend to have few reserves to deal with additional stress and decompensate easily and generally avoid stressful situations, whereas people with low levels of basal anxiety tend to seek anxiety-provoking situations for pleasure. The former (e.g. librarians and clerks) avoid stress as much as possible and thrive on calm order; the latter (e.g. motor cycle racers) enjoy taking risks (Fig. 4.2).

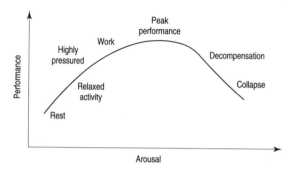

Fig. 4.2 The Yerkes Dodson curve. (From Yerkes R, Dodson J 1908. The relation of strength of a stimulus to rapidity of habit-formation. Journal of Comparative and Neurological Psychology 18:459–482.)

4.11

What determines individual responses to stressors?

In general, individuals can probably cope with most stressful situations providing they are desensitized to them gradually. Most people can learn to overcome the stress of a situation, such as public speaking, with practice and habituation. Added to this are factors such as the innate ability to respond to anxiety-provoking situations and the ability to habituate. In addition, the significance of any event, such as losing a job, depends on the personal circumstances: a man or woman with a family and mortgage to support will experience far more stress than an individual with no commitment who feels the need for a change in any case. Some events are more stressful than others if there has been less opportunity to prepare for them emotionally, or if demands are made which are well beyond personal capability, or if they are unpredictable and unfamiliar.

4.12

What can be done to help overcome depression in the people who look after and care for the elderly or mentally and physically disabled?

It is easy to overlook the contribution of carers to the well-being of their dependants and focus simply on the needs of the notional patient. Carers often have an ambivalent attitude to their charge, on one hand feeling a sense of duty, and on the other hand having a desire for freedom. These conflicting emotions often result in internal conflict and stress. Carers should be encouraged to attend support groups and to join the Care Attenders Scheme, which can give them the afternoon off from time to time. Listening, and trying to help them with their practical needs, is important. Respite care should be arranged. Services such as the home incontinence laundry are helpful. Where appropriate, there should be referral to the domiciliary occupational therapy services to make adaptations in the home.

4.13

What is burn-out? What signs should we be looking for in our colleagues, and how should it be treated?

Burn-out is a condition which occurs in people doing too stressful jobs for too long. People try hard but are continually thwarted in their attempt to succeed. After a period of time people become frustrated and indifferent. It is an occupational hazard of health-care professionals and educationalists, often affecting the more enthusiastic and energetic.

It can be recognized by increasing irritability at work and loss of interest. Burn-out victims are exhausted physically, emotionally and attitudinally. They start making mistakes and develop coping strategies such as drinking or avoidance of work. More subtle variants are seen in people who pick holes in their colleagues' work, and who become hypercritical of the management structures.

It is important to recognize this condition before it becomes chronic and, ideally, to arrange for a change in working conditions, or at least a prolonged holiday. Counselling may be helpful and attention to adequate diversionary and recreationary activities is important.

4.14

How can we help our patients decrease and manage their own stress?

It is helpful to advise patients to set realistic goals and to structure their time wisely between work, family and recreation. They might benefit from a short course of counselling sessions which would enable them to share their burdens and is often quite helpful.

The use of excessive alcohol, smoking and drugs should be avoided. Patients should be encouraged to take exercise and use relaxation techniques such as self-hypnosis, which can be learned from tapes, or by joining stress groups run by a practice counsellor. It may be useful to separate patients with established anxiety symptoms from those who are suffering from the pressures of life. A stress clinic run within the surgery can be used to teach relaxation techniques, and to offer simple counselling. Some people favour the use of techniques such as autogenic training, which is a variant of anxiety management, but focuses away from the concept of disease into more healthy living.

ADVERSE LIFE EVENTS

4.15

When should symptoms of anxiety or depression, arising as a consequence of an adverse life event, be treated?

Bereavements and loss, including adverse life events such as divorce, redundancy and homelessness, classically result in symptoms of depression, whereas the anticipation of loss and stress precipitates anxiety symptoms. In most cases this is an appropriate response. The psyche has great powers of adaptation, and in general individuals learn and profit from dealing with adverse circumstances. A certain degree of suffering is unavoidable and learning to cope with it properly is a part of life. Adverse life events can also trigger episodes of major psychiatric illness, which can then run on independently of the underlying cause, even if it is resolved. The question of when to treat depends upon the severity of the illness and the symptoms as well as their duration. Tranquillizers and hypnotics pose a particular problem because they block habituation and learning. Therefore, if there is a real external stressor which requires the individual to adapt, prescribing benzodiazepines will possibly impair that adaptive process. This is not to say that distressing symptoms which last more than a week or so after an adverse event should not be treated, for example, prescribing one or two nights' benzodiazepine hypnotic for insomnia. This is not medicalizing a normal situation, if it is what the patient requests. As a rule of thumb, normal grief reactions can last up to a year, and if they last longer, patients should be treated with antidepressants or anxiolytics. There is no reason why medication cannot be introduced sooner if the symptoms are so disabling as significantly to impair functioning. There is no benefit in prolonging suffering when adequate treatment may be available. This is especially so in acute post-traumatic stress disorders, when experience shows that sedation over a week or so may be the treatment of choice before returning the individual to normal functioning after a major occurrence, such as battle stress or a natural disaster.

4.16

How can normal grief be distinguished from grief and depression which may need active treatment?

Grief and a certain amount of depression are normal after the loss of a close relative or friend. Some degree of distress is inevitable, but if the distress continually interferes with the individual's life and lasts for a period of several months, active treatment should be instituted. All bereaved individuals may benefit from simple counselling and empathetic contact with another individual who has had similar experiences, and from an opportunity to ventilate their feelings, as well as from involvement in social activities.

4.17

Are there factors which predispose to serious grief reactions?

Grief reactions are worse after sudden and unexpected bereavement. They are most protracted after ambivalent relationships where the bereaved was in a situation of conflict, and, despite emotional involvement, also wished ill to the deceased. Such relationships often result in guilt. Intense yearning following the death is most pronounced when the bereaved was dependent on the former spouse and needed help in basic activities of daily living.

4.18

What can be done to help the recently bereaved patient?

Bereaved people need to talk about the deceased and their relationship, the illness, the mode of death and the funeral. They need to be allowed to ventilate the anger, guilt and frustration they feel. Brief counselling and contact with bereavement groups are appropriate. Severe, prolonged and pathological depression should be treated with antidepressants, and short-term anxiety and insomnia may benefit from anxiolytics and sleeping pills for a few days.

Good social support from the family and neighbours is helpful in minimizing grief reactions. Feelings of self-worth are increased in the bereaved with jobs, careers and new relationships and are helpful for reducing grief reactions.

4.19

What evidence is there to link depression and unemployment?

Employment provides structure, worth, self-esteem and finance, as well as channelling creative drives. In general, providing work is not overstressful, it enhances mental well-being. Unemployment is associated with an increased risk of emotional distress, depression and depressive illnesses of varying degrees of severity. The scientific evidence linking unemployment and depression has methodological flaws since many people with mental problems are likely to be unemployed, but in general unemployment leads to depression and also to increased suicide rates.

4.20

What are the symptoms of post-traumatic stress disorder?

This is quite a common condition in minor forms after, for example, an accident or assault. It is more severe after a person has experienced an event that is outside the range of usual human experience and would be markedly distressing to almost anyone – for example, a serious threat to one's life or harm to one's children or community. It is characterized by a series of symptoms such as recurrent and intrusive memories of the event, distressing dreams, flashbacks and intense psychological distress when the memories of the event are triggered. There are efforts to avoid thoughts or feelings associated with the trauma and the person develops feelings of detachment with regard to others. It is associated with irritability and other symptoms of anxiety.

4.21

How should post-traumatic stress disorder be treated?

In the acute stages, sedation is the treatment of choice. It is then treated by guided imagery, allowing the individuals to relive the event and explore their feelings in a controlled situation over a period of time. Otherwise the condition is treated symptomatically according to which particular symptoms are most obvious and distressing. This may include both pharmacological and psychological treatment as appropriate.

COPING MECHANISMS

4.22

Why do more women than men take tranquillizers?

First of all, women tend to consult their GP more than men about a wide range of problems, including anxiety and depression, and are therefore more likely to be given tranquillizers. Interestingly, women GPs are more likely to prescribe tranquillizers than their male colleagues. The sociological view would be that women are encouraged to adopt dependent roles in society, and dependency on benzodiazepines is just a variant on this. Also, it is seen as more acceptable for women to take tranquillizers, and men to drink. Both are mechanisms for reducing anxiety.

4.23

What proportion of anxious patients self-medicate with alcohol?

Twice as many women as men consume tranquillizers and the corollary is that men drink alcohol instead. Thus, half of the anxious men will drink alcohol, and half will take anxiolytics. Anecdotal evidence shows that many alcoholics embarked upon a career of heavy drinking as a form of self-medication for anxiety states. Alcohol is, of course, widely used as a social lubricant to deal with minor normal insecurities at social gatherings and has been said to make 'social intercourse possible and sometimes even palatable'.

However, alcohol is a poor anxiolytic. Tolerance to its effects develops rapidly and consumption increases. Soon people drink from habit and become drunk before the anxiolytic effects occur. Alcohol is also quite a toxic substance and cannot be recommended for more than occasional anxiolysis.

4.24

How can the problems of alcoholism be untangled from any underlying depression?

Alcoholism, anxiety and depression are closely linked. Many alcoholics start drinking to excess to relieve chronic symptoms of depression or, more commonly, anxiety or for 'Dutch courage'. By the time the problem gets out of hand they have often forgotten why they started to drink. There is also a statistical, and possibly genetic, link between depression and alcoholism. Unfortunately, after several years' established drinking, the underlying pathology becomes blurred. Most alcoholics are really quite low when drinking, but after a couple of days of abstinence feel remarkably better until the next crisis comes along and they start drinking again. For someone who is drinking heavily, there is no alternative to abstinence before a proper assessment can be made. In patients drinking moderate amounts the distinction can be more difficult.

4.25

Is there any evidence that nicotine has an anxiolytic effect?

Nicotine is both anxiolytic and anxiogenic. This appears to be a function of dose and probably individual variability. There is also an aspect of learned behaviour, in that smokers have learned to interpret the effects of nicotine as anxiolytic. There is also a strong behavioural effect associated with the ritual of having a break and a cigarette.

4.26

Why is the avoidance practised by some patients with anxiety disorders counter-productive? Surely it is sensible to avoid that which provokes the anxiety?

Avoidance in simple phobias, such as of snakes, spiders and other specific situations or objects, is quite common and probably normal. In most cases, avoidance of the specific stimulus is not necessarily harmful. Unfortunately, in more severe phobias, the fear is generally excessive, and, once triggered, avoidance tends to generalize. The important point is to deal with avoidant behaviour at an early stage before this can happen. For example, a fear of committing a social blunder in public can lead to a severe limitation on social life. Thus, what is a simple fear of one situation can extend into other situations as well. If the phobia is not confronted early on, retreat from the fear becomes an established reaction; then as the condition develops, avoidance becomes worse, ultimately becoming disabling and limiting. In the milder forms, patients develop elaborate rituals to avoid specific situations; in its worst form agoraphobics can be become housebound for many years and severely limit their enjoyment of normal life.

5 SPECIAL GROUPS

Introduction

Certain ethnic groups are more likely to suffer from severe depressions than others. For example, depression is more common among Jewish people. Severe and recurrent depressions affect men and women in equal proportions where genetic factors seem important.

Milder depression is more common among women, and vulnerability factors include low socio-economic status, three or more children under the age of 14, lack of a confiding relationship with husband or partner, and lack of employment. It is hardly surprising that these are associated with significant depression. Early loss of mother (before the age of 11) also seems to predispose to depression, presumably giving rise to developmental problems as a result of a lack of adequate modelling. The elderly, children and those with physical illnesses are also at particular risk of developing depression and anxiety for several reasons. These vulnerability factors predispose to mild to moderate depression.

DEPRESSION IN WOMEN

5.1

Is the incidence of anxiety higher in women than in men?

Anxiety disorders are probably as common in men as in women, but women tend to present to their GP about twice as frequently with anxiety symptoms as do men. This is true across a wide variety of complaints, not only in the psychological spectrum.

The reasons for this are complex. It is generally more acceptable for women to complain about themselves than men, who are expected to be more stoical. Women tend to seek medical solutions for their symptoms, whereas men reduce their anxiety levels by drinking alcohol.

Biological factors may also be relevant since progesterone and its metabolites act on the benzodiazepine receptor complex. This may account for variations in mood associated with the menstrual cycle.

5.2

Is the incidence of depression higher in women than in men?

Men and women suffer severe bipolar disorder equally, but, overall, depression appears to affect women about twice as much as men. This is not simply due to women reporting distress or seeking help more than men. It is known that depression is particularly high in women in socio-economic group 5 who live in isolated and deprived circumstances, bringing up children without adequate support. On the other hand, there is also a high incidence in socio-economic group 1. It has been suggested that middle-class women are particularly vulnerable to feelings of guilt, low self-esteem and depression, which they use to express their sense of personal failure. It appears biologists, sociologists and psychologists can find suitable models that explain the statistics to support their own viewpoint.

5.3

What factors predispose to stress-related illness in women?

Several stressful factors can be identified (see Box 5.1).

Box 5.1   FACTORS PREDISPOSING TO STRESS-RELATED ILLNESS IN WOMEN

- Being a mother under 20 with several young children under five
- Poor relations with partner
- Health problems
- Financial worries
- Housing problems
- Poor sleeping and tiredness
- Busy job and trying to run a home
- Premenstrual tension
- Difficult, wilful and argumentative children
- Unemployment/redundancy
- Death of a close friend.

5.4

Is there any relationship between premenstrual tension (PMT) and depression?

There is a considerable overlap between the symptoms of PMT and depression. At a biochemical level, brain 5-HT systems appear to be blunted premenstrually, and antidepressants can relieve premenstrual symptoms. Progestogens can also have an effect on the benzodiazepine receptor, and benzodiazepines can relieve PMT. On a psychological level, women with a tendency to depression are more likely to suffer from, or notice, the symptoms of PMT. In general if women are feeling happy and robust, it is easier to ignore or deal with painful breasts, irritability and other aspects of the syndrome.

5.5

Is there a place for counselling for women after miscarriage?

Many women become very depressed after a miscarriage and often feel unable to talk about it as it is not a socially acceptable subject for discussion like pregnancy. Most of these women are seen and treated in general practice by sympathetic listening, and sometimes bereavement counselling. They often feel they have failed in their primary role as women and are terrified that they will never conceive again and deliver a baby. Repeated miscarriage can place enormous strains on both partners, yet while the physical issues are often addressed by obstetricians, few people pay attention to the emotional problems associated with miscarriage. It can be helpful for women to come into contact with other women who have had similar problems, since miscarriages are so frequent, and it helps women to realize they are not unique or failures. A helpful book might be *Miscarriage* by Ann Oakley. Ultimately, the best treatment is to become pregnant again and have a fine, healthy baby.

5.6

How common is postnatal depression?

'Post-baby blues' is probably a normal reaction affecting the majority of mothers in the first few days following childbirth. Postnatal depression affects maybe 10 to 15% of all women in the first postnatal year, but frank puerperal psychosis occurs in only one or two women per thousand deliveries. 'Porridge brain', a condition when women are unable to think clearly, concentrate properly or have their normal energy, is quite common and almost normal in the first year after childbirth.

5.7

What are the symptoms of postnatal depression?

The clinical features are essentially those of neurotic depression with anxiety and irritability as well. Tearfulness and tiredness contribute to a feeling of general inadequacy. There is poor concentration, loss of appetite and sleep disturbance may also be present. Loss of libido is often profound, and may exacerbate a strained marital relationship. Vague physical symptoms such as headache, backache and vaginal discharge without obvious cause are common. Obsessional thoughts about harming the baby may be present, and very occasionally women may feel suicidal. The condition may occur at any time in the first year after childbirth, and can vary in severity from quite severe illness to a relatively mild condition bordering on the normal.

5.8

Is it possible to predict which mothers will develop postnatal depression?

Women with higher levels of depressive symptoms during pregnancy and a history of previous episodes of depression or a history of premenstrual depression are at increased risk for the blues. A family history of depression is also associated with increased risk. Stress during the pregnancy may be instrumental in turning the post-baby blues into a postnatal depression.

5.9

Is there a suitable screening test to help identify postnatal depression?

The Edinburgh Postnatal Depression Scale is a screening test which helps identify mothers at risk of significant postnatal depression (Fig. 5.1).

As you have recently had a baby, we would like to know how you are feeling.
Please **circle the score** that comes closest to how you have felt IN THE PAST 7 DAYS, not just how you feel today. Here is an example, already completed.

1. I have felt happy:
0   Yes, all the time
(1)   Yes, most of the time
2   No, not very often
3   No, not at all

This would mean: 'I have felt happy most of the time' during the past week. Please complete the other questions in the same way:

Fig. 5.1 Edinburgh Postnatal Depression Scale. (From Cox J, Holden J, Sagovsky R 1987. Detection of postnatal depression. British Journal of Psychiatry 150:782–786.)

In the past 7 days

1. I have been able to laugh and see the funny side of things:
0 As much as I always could
1 Not quite so much now
2 Definitely not so much now
3 Not at all

2. I have looked forward with enjoyment to things:
0 As much as I ever did
1 Rather less than I used to
2 Definitely less than I used to
3 Hardly at all

*3. I have blamed myself unnecessarily when things went wrong:
3 Yes, most of the time
2 Yes, some of the time
1 Not very often
0 No, never

4. I have been anxious or worried for no good reason:
0 No, not at all
1 Hardly ever
2 Yes, sometimes
3 Yes, very often

*5. I have felt scared or panicky for no very good reason:
3 Yes, quite a lot
2 Yes, sometimes
1 No, not much
0 No, not at all

*6. Things have been getting on top of me:
3 Yes, most of the time I haven't been able to cope at all
2 Yes, sometimes I haven't been coping as well as usual
1 No, most of the time I have coped quite well
0 No, I have been coping as well as ever

*7. I have been so unhappy that I have had difficulty sleeping:
3 Yes, most of the time
2 Yes, sometimes
1 Not very often
0 No, not at all

*8. I have felt sad or miserable:
3 Yes, most of the time
2 Yes, quite often
1 Not very often
0 No, not at all

*9. I have been so unhappy that I have been crying:
3 Yes, most of the time
2 Yes, quite often
1 Only occasionally
0 No, never

*10. The thought of harming myself has occurred to me:
3 Yes, quite often
2 Sometimes
1 Hardly ever
0 Never

Instructions for users

The mother is asked to circle the response that comes closest to how she has been feeling in the previous 7 days.

All ten items must be completed.

Care should be taken to avoid the possibility of the mother discussing her answers with others.

The mother should complete the scale herself, unless she has limited English or has difficulty with reading.

The EPDS may be used at 6–8 weeks to screen postnatal women. The child health clinic, postnatal check-up or a home visit may provide suitable opportunities for completion.

Response categories are scored 0, 1, 2 and 3 according to increased severity of the symptoms, items marked with an asterisk are reverse scored (3, 2, 1 and 0). The total score is calculated by adding together the scores for each of the ten items.

Mothers who score above a threshold of 12/13 are likely to be suffering from a depressive illness of varying severity.

For routine use in primary care, it might be appropriate to assess further those mothers scoring above a threshold of 9/10.

The score should not override clinical judgement, and a careful clinical assessment should be carried out to confirm the diagnosis.

The scale indicates how the mother has felt during the previous week, and in doubtful cases it may be usefully repeated after 2 weeks.

The scale will not detect mothers with anxiety neuroses, phobias or personality disorders.

Fig. 5.1 *(cont'd)*

5.10

What can help prevent postnatal depression?

When reviewing women at an antenatal clinic, those at risk, either because of social problems or because of previous episodes, can be identified. By establishing an avenue of communication, women at risk of postnatal depression can be monitored better and are more likely to present problems should they arise. This may not prevent postnatal depression, but it does facilitate prompt detection and treatment should the condition develop.

5.11

How serious is postnatal psychosis and what steps should be taken to safeguard the new baby?

Postnatal psychosis can involve suicidal thinking and neglect of the baby. It is a very rare disorder and is usually detected early. Some mothers develop obsessional fears of harming their baby, but this arises out of their desire to do the best rather than wishing the baby ill, and is not in itself dangerous. Most depressive states are not directly harmful to the baby, although the mother may be fearful of letting health care professionals know, in the mistaken belief that her child may be taken away. Postnatal psychosis usually has a good prognosis, but may require admission to a psychiatric unit, ideally with a mother and baby facility, although these are not widely available. Rarely, it may be the start of a chronic psychotic illness. Social Services should be involved early if there is a suspicion that the baby is at risk. Foster parents can be found if necessary, while the mother recovers. Unfortunately, I see increasing numbers of schizophrenic mothers, in unstable relationships who have children without the real ability to look after them. We then become involved in the agonizing business of helping a court to decide whether the child should be taken away from them or not.

5.12

Is there a relationship between the menopause and depression?

Although social and hormonal factors may have a part to play in involutional melancholia, depressive illnesses have a natural tendency to occur later in life. The symptoms of the menopause should be treated and hormone replacement therapy (HRT) given as appropriate. Counselling may be offered. Whatever the cause of the depressive symptoms, it may be worth treating them with antidepressants if the symptoms warrant it.

5.13

How does HRT affect depression?

HRT improves psychological well-being and relieves irritability, fatigue, anxiety and depression. It has been reported to cause depression, but this is uncommon. HRT by itself is not sufficient to treat depression in postmenopausal women, but may help improve general well-being in milder forms of depression.

CHILDREN AND ADOLESCENTS

5.14

Are anxiety and depression distinguishable in children?

The classification of mood disorders is even more imprecise in childhood than in adults. There is considerable overlap between anxiety, depression and other disorders in children. The cardinal feature of depressive disorders in this age group is the lack of the ability to have fun and play. Normal children make a game of most things, whereas depressed children isolate themselves and do not become involved in things going on around them.

5.15

How does anxiety present in children?

Anxiety presents in several different ways. Children may develop somatic symptoms without obvious physical cause apart from physiological arousal. They may have sleep disturbance with insomnia and nightmares. They may regress to a younger emotional level, adopting more childlike behaviour, such as uncharacteristic bed-wetting or soiling and poor work or school performance due to impaired concentration. They may also develop obsessional symptoms. Some anxieties may be persistent, and others appear only when the child is exposed to a specific fear situation such as school, resulting in school refusal. Physiologically there may be headaches, abdominal pain, tachycardia, hyperventilation, sweating, tremor, pallor, vomiting and pains due to muscle tension.

5.16

How should children with anxiety disorders be treated?

If the causes of the child's anxiety are relatively straightforward and obvious, such as bullying at school or problems in the home, the parents should be counselled on how to deal with the situation, for example, by discussing the problem with the teachers in the case of bullying, or by taking steps to resolve their conflicts if there is marital disharmony. If the causation of the anxiety is less obvious or harder to deal with, then referral to a specialist is appropriate. The usual line of treatment would be along psychological lines, exploring the causation of the symptoms. This often needs to be done in a family interview. Anxiolytic medication is rarely indicated and should be within the province of the specialist.

5.17

How common is depression in childhood?

Approximately 10% of 10-year-olds report symptoms of misery and unhappiness, but depressive syndromes occur in less than 2% of children and 4% of adolescents. Full-blown depressive illnesses occur in 0.15% of 10-year-olds and 1.5% of 14-year-olds. In outpatients at child psychiatry units, up to 25% of children will be depressed; about half of inpatients will have depressive disorders. It is more common among boys than girls before puberty, and more common among girls after puberty. Overall, depression is rare before puberty and has a similar incidence to that in adults after puberty. Mania is also rare before puberty. Presumably hormonal factors are important in the expression of mood disorder.

5.18

What factors might contribute to, or be the cause of a child becoming depressed?

Children generally respond to problems in their environment. They become depressed as a result of loss – for example, the death of a parent or grandparent – or divorce. They may be subject to bullying in school, or suffer from poor performance as a result of undiagnosed dyslexia, deafness or other learning impairments. If one parent is depressed, children can often develop depressive patterns of behaviour, either because of learned helplessness, or possibly because of some genetic influence. Children may become depressed as a result of excessive responsibility in the family, and, most importantly, because of sexual or physical abuse. Problems in the home, such as rows, financial difficulties or unemployment, also contribute to depression in children.

5.19

How can depression be assessed in children?

Many children are too young to realize they feel depressed or to be able to describe their feelings. The important thing is to gather information from many different sources, including the child, the parents and possible community contacts such as school teachers. Many children present with depressive symptoms, but their parents are unaware of their significance, although a history needs to be taken from the parents. Children may manifest behavioural problems: poor performance at school, school avoidance, bed-wetting and nightmares.

The child may display feelings of loss, disappointment and sadness, aggressive behaviour, general disenchantment and lack of caring. Depressed children lose interest in play and lack enjoyment in life.

5.20

How is depression treated in children?

Some children have clear depressive illnesses which are clinically indistinguishable from those described in adults. They may have a classical agitated depression and respond to antidepressant drugs, which are the treatment of choice over other forms of therapy. There is a larger group of depressed children whose problems are related to life difficulties, for whom the treatment is dealing with, and helping them to come to terms with, their difficulties. These are usually to do with problems, often arising in the children themselves, or within the family. A third group of children presents with anti-social or conduct disorders, school failure and drug abuse. These are all symptoms secondary to depression, although the presentation is part of bad behaviour. (Not all children with conduct disorder are depressed.)

The standard approach to assessing and treating depression in children is by using a multidisciplinary team of child and family psychiatrists as well as child psychologists, social workers and educationalists. Treatment is along psychosocial lines. Treatment with antidepressants is generally regarded as no better than placebo, although both treatments make substantial improvements. There are very few adequate studies to address the place of antidepressants in children.

5.21

What factors contribute to the development of depression in adolescents?

In many ways, the same factors are at work that contribute to depression in children. Puberty, however, has a part to play in increasing the risk, and the prevalence of depressive disorders rises to a level comparable with that of adults. Thus, pressures at school for exams, career choices and possible unemployment are important, as are the pressures to succeed and conform and other peer pressures.

The emergence of more adult emotions and sexual feelings may be difficult to deal with. Sexual abuse is a powerful disturber of self-worth and an important possible factor to consider. In adolescent development, there comes a time when some decide they will not succeed in normal adult endeavours and determine to adopt peer morals and social deviancy. It is important to note that adolescence is also a time when anorexia nervosa and schizophrenia begin to manifest themselves.

5.22

What specific questions can I ask to help me diagnose depression in this age group?

A useful mnemonic device is HEADSSS:

HEADSSS
• H Homes – can you talk to your parents?
• E Education – ask for actual marks
• A Activities – ask about friends
• D Drugs – are they being abused?
• S Sex – is this a problem?
• S Suicide – consider the risk
• S Sleep – look for sleep disturbance

Changes in appetite, either increasing or decreasing, should be noted as should loss of interest in activities that are usually found enjoyable, such as sports and social activities. It is important to look for the signs of profound social withdrawal.

5.23

Are suicide rates rising in this age group?

The real suicide rate is increasing, particularly in boys between the ages of 15 and 20. This is in marked contrast to all other age groups, apart from elderly males, where the suicide rate is gradually reducing. Adolescent boys are at particular risk of violent death, accidents as well as suicide. Having once made a suicide attempt, the risk of a further attempt is about 50%. A family history of suicidal behaviour is common among children and adolescents who attempt suicide.

THE ELDERLY

5.24

How common is depression in the elderly?

A quarter of people over the age of 65 have some depressive symptoms. Most depressive illnesses in this group can be diagnosed as dysphoria of old age, related more to social isolation and adverse life events, such as bereavement. In over half of the over-65s, minor depression is associated with concomitant physical illness rather than primary depressive disorder.

More serious depression is found in about 10% of this group and about 5% have severe depression which warrants referral to a specialist.

5.25

How does depression present in elderly patients in nursing homes?

It may be difficult to recognize depression in patients over 75 years of age, especially those who live in an institution. One-third of people in residential care have been shown to be depressed. It is always a possibility. Does the resident look tense and gloomy and feel worried or is the resident complacent about his or her symptoms? Is there a loss of interest in the surrounding environment and a change in sleep pattern? Does the patient assess past life and achievements pessimistically? Does the future hold any hope, or would he or she rather be dead? Diurnal variation in mood is particularly important, as are symptoms of loss of memory and concentration, and a fear of dementia as well as physical self-neglect.

Some patients show agitated depression, whereas others have slowness of thought.

5.26

What measures should be taken to prevent the development of depression in the elderly?

Old age is associated with changes in circumstances and bereavements, often loss of one's spouse, career and disposable income, sexual potency, and so on. It is not surprising that many elderly people feel depressed. The most important thing is pre-retirement planning, and counselling, especially in relation to financial matters and pensions, which cannot be begun too early. Alternatives to paid employment should be explored. Sexual dysfunction should be treated where appropriate. Incontinence can be particularly troublesome and may need treatment, possibly surgically. The possibility of thyroid dysfunction as well as other significant medical problems should be considered. Mental and physical activity are important to health and voluntary work and regular exercise are pathways to this. A good diet and social life also encourage well-being. From a medical point of view, you should consider HRT in women if appropriate. Bereavement counselling is also important.

5.27

What is the best treatment for depression in the elderly?

There is a strong case to be made for prescribing the newer antidepressants (SSRIs, serotonin noradrenergic reuptake inhibitors (SNRIs) or lofepramine) in this group, ideally at lower doses, or MAOIs, which are also effective. If simple measures fail, ECT should be considered. It is often highly effective in this group and the side effects and safety of this treatment are probably less of a drawback in the elderly than the effects of oral medication.

5.28

What are the specific problems associated with the use of antidepressants in the elderly?

The elderly have an increased sensitivity to the side effects of drugs, and with a low body mass they need a much lower dosage, possibly a third of the adult dose of standard antidepressants. Concomitant disease, dementia and poor compliance add to the difficulties in prescribing. Specifically, cardiotoxicity of older antidepressants, resulting from the quinidine-like and alpha-blocking action of some antidepressants, is a problem. Constipation, prostatism and glaucoma are adversely affected by the anticholinergic action, which may impair memory function, too, and the antihistamine actions impede psychomotor function.

5.29

How should dosage be determined for antidepressant therapy?

When prescribing antidepressants in the elderly, it is best to start off at a low dose before gradually titrating upwards: 'start low and go slow'.

5.30

I find it even more difficult to diagnose depression where there is a degree of senile dementia present as well. Presumably treating the depression may improve the overall mental state. How can I differentiate between the two conditions and decide who to treat?

There are many similarities between dementia and pseudo-dementia, which is a depressive state mimicking dementia. The most obvious way to tell the two conditions apart is by assessing the patient's memory. In depression patients will simply say 'I don't know' if they can't answer the question, whereas demented patients will either confabulate (make up appropriate answers), or perseverate (repeat the question or the answer several times). Demented patients also have visuospatial difficulties which can be detected by making them draw a clock face or other complex diagram. A score of less than 25 on a mini-mental state test is likely to be diagnostic of dementia (Fig. 5.2).

		Maximum score	Patients actual score

Now I would like to ask some questions to check your concentration and your memory.
Most of them will be easy. *Score zero for refusal, error or can't do. Enter ticks in the appropriate boxes*

ORIENTATION

What is the ...   year?   season?   month?   date?   day of the week?   **(5)**

Do you know what .... room we are in?
floor we are on?
street we are in?   **(5)**
town we are in?
city/county we are in?

REGISTRATION

I am going to name three objects. After I have said them, I want you to repeat them. Remember what they are because I am going to ask you to repeat them again in a few minutes.   **(3)**

Please repeat the three items for me ...... 'APPLE' ... 'TABLE' ... 'PENNY' ...
Score first try. Repeat objects until all are learnt.

ATTENTION AND CALCULATION

D	
L	
R	**(5)**
O	
W	

Now I am going to spell a word forwards and I want you to spell it backwards. The word is WORLD. W – O – R – L – D. Spell 'world' backwards.
Repeat if necessary but not after spelling starts. Record spelling opposite.
Score 1 point for each letter in the correct position e.g. dlrow = 5; dlorw = 3.

RECALL

Ask the patient if he can recall the three objects repeated above.   **(3)**
Score 1 point for each correct answer.

LANGUAGE

Naming   Show the patient a wrist watch and ask him what it is.
e.g. 'What is this called?' Repeat for a pencil.   **(2)**

Repetition   Ask the patient to repeat the following sentence after you.
'NO IFS, ANDS OR BUTS' *Allow only one trial.*

Follow a 3-stage command Give the patient a piece of plain blank paper and repeat the command. *Score 1 point for each part correctly executed.*

Fig. 5.2 Mini-mental state examination which is read out by doctors.

	'Take a paper in your right hand, fold the paper in half with both hands and put it on the floor'	(3)	
Reading	Show the patient the piece of paper provided with the sentence 'Close your eyes' printed in letters large enough for the patient to see clearly. Ask him to read it and do what it says. *Score 1 point only if he actually closes his eyes.*		
	Read and obey the following:		
	CLOSE YOUR EYES	(1)	
Writing	Give the patient a blank piece of paper and ask him to write a sentence for you. Do not dictate a sentence, it has to be written spontaneously. It must contain a subject and verb and be sensible. Correct grammer and punctuation are not necessary.		
	Write a sentence	(1)	
Copying	Present the patient with the intersecting pentagon design, and ask him to copy it exactly as it is. All 10 angles must be present and 2 must intersect to score 1 point. Tremor and rotation are ignored.		
	Copy design in the space provided.	(1)	

Fig. 5.2 *(cont'd)*

5.31

Is an element of anxiety always present in dementia?

Many patients in the advance stages of dementia have no symptoms of anxiety. Anxiety is often present in the early stages of the illness when patients realize they are developing problems with their memory, and this in itself is anxiety provoking. In cases of established dementia, anxiety may be a feature, presumably as a result of the underlying pathological process, or as part of a depressive syndrome or agitation.

5.32

How should insomnia be treated in the elderly?

The elderly do sleep less, but it is a generalization to say that they all sleep badly. The inability to sleep through the night is distressing and is

93

a major reason why patients seek medication. Sleep hygiene involves no cat-napping during the day, as much stimulation as possible during waking hours, and appropriate physical exercise, avoiding cups of tea or coffee prior to sleeping, and dealing with problems such as pain or intercurrent illness. It is important not to miss a depressive illness as a cause of sleep disturbance. If it is appropriate to prescribe a hypnotic, it is advisable to avoid long-acting benzodiazepines because of hangovers and falls. Zopiclone is a reasonable choice, and a sedative tricyclic or trazodone may be appropriate if depression is present.

CONCOMITANT CONDITIONS

5.33

Should patients who seem to have depressive symptoms associated with physical illness be referred to a psychiatrist?

Many people with physical illnesses also have depressive symptoms, and depressive symptoms may well make the expression of physical illness and the resultant morbidity worse. Thus, the two are closely interlinked. Deciding the proportion of blame attached to the physical problem and the psychological component in this circular condition can be difficult. Psychiatrists are used to seeing patients with severe depression, and are less good at dealing with milder disorders. GPs recognize milder symptoms as important in depression. In milder depression (dysphoria), which psychiatrists are not good at treating, it is often difficult to decide at which level to start treating since we know antidepressants usually do not work in this form of depression, and the counselling and support on offer are probably directed at dealing with psychological and functional disability associated with physical illness.

5.34

Does depression affect the prognosis of serious disease?

As many as 20% of patients with long-standing physical illness may also suffer from significant depression. The depressive symptoms can be difficult to distinguish from those of the physical illness. The factors determining exactly which patients will develop depression are not clear, and are not dependent upon any specific illness or patient variables. Taking the example of breast cancer, about a quarter of women suffer significant depression, anxiety and sexual dysfunction after mastectomy, and the risk is increased in those with poor marital relationships, unsupportive social networks, recent adverse life events and previous psychiatric illness. Despite this, very few are referred to a psychiatrist. Many who experience psychological reactions respond well to brief interventions, such as one or two counselling sessions, or group interventions, including relaxation training and supportive psychotherapy. This approach shows beneficial effects on depression, anxiety and physical symptoms such as pain, as well as general well-being. Some works suggest that a fighting spirit helps patients live longer, and adverse life events may be associated with relapses. Some studies have shown that psychotherapy in patients with advanced breast cancer can prolong life. Nevertheless, the suggestion that the course of the cancer itself can be affected by the treatment of depression, remains speculative.

5.35

What treatment should be offered to a middle-aged asthmatic lady who is excessively anxious about everything?

Breathless patients are often quite anxious as well, partly because it is extremely worrying having to fight for every breath of air. Studies have shown that reducing anxiety levels can also improve pulmonary function. The level of breathlessness in chronic obstructive airways disease is not determined purely by the diameter of the bronchial lumen, but by the level of anxiety as well. Reducing anxiety improves breathlessness. The matter is further complicated by the fact that many patients who complain of breathlessness are actually hyperventilating as a feature of their anxiety state.

Treatment options include counselling and psychotherapy, to explore issues of how it feels to be breathless, and an element of cognitive therapy to explore the psychological implications of breathlessness for the patient.

Beta-blockers are contraindicated because they may cause bronchospasm. Benzodiazepines may induce dependence if used long term and can reduce respiratory drive if the patient is hypercapnoeic.

Non-benzodiazepine anxiolytics such as buspirone are useful in the treatment of anxiety symptoms in breathless patients.

5.36

How common is depression after a stroke?

Emotional disturbance and misery are common after a stroke and depression is more common than in the general population. Anxiety is common and is best dealt with by explanation and support.

It is difficult to assess the extent of any depressive illness in a patient who has had a stroke, possibly because of the facial paralysis and speech problems as well as emotional lability which may co-exist.

5.37

How should depression following a stroke be treated?

It is important to attend to the patient's social and psychological, as well as psychiatric, needs and this may involve dealing with problems of incontinence, mobility and social isolation, as well as pharmacological treatment for the depression. Elderly patients may have co-existent Parkinson's disease, and others may have widespread vascular disease, so it is probably better to use one of the more modern antidepressants rather than sedative tricyclics. If in doubt, it is worth giving a therapeutic trial of an antidepressant.

5.38

How should depression in patients with Parkinson's disease be treated?

Anxiety and depression are quite common in these patients. The difficulty in making a diagnosis or assessment of depression is compounded by the paucity of facial expression. The most obvious way to assess depression is to ask patients how they feel. Unfortunately, antidepressants are not very effective in this condition. Because of the abnormality of dopamine metabolism, it is probably worth using a broad-spectrum antidepressant such as lofepramine. It should be remembered that anti-Parkinsonian agents can also cause a disturbed mental state and the effective treatment of the Parkinson's disease may also improve mood.

5.39

What is the role of tricyclic antidepressants in the treatment of severe chronic pain?

It appears tricyclic antidepressants have a specific pain-relieving action, especially on peripheral neuropathic pain. This is independent of their antidepressant action. They often work in much lower doses than is necessary for their antidepressant effect. Drugs such as clomipramine and imipramine or dothiepine, given at 20 or 50 mg daily, are regarded as helpful by pain specialists. There is some evidence to suggest that they act by increasing brain endorphin levels. They may also have an inherent analgesic effect. The pain threshold may also be increased by treating any associated depression. SSRIs appear to be less helpful.

5.40

Should patients with irritable bowel syndrome (IBS) be treated symptomatically for the bowel disorder or should they be given treatment for the anxiety and/or depression and hope that the gut symptom will improve as well?

The primary treatment of IBS should be directed at the bowel with antispasmodics and guidance on diet. Many of these patients are referred to a psychiatrist with relatively mild anxiety or depressive syndromes, and for them antidepressants are less effective. If symptoms are significant, it may be appropriate to prescribe an antidepressant. The older tricyclics have an anticholinergic action which may be unhelpful. The new SSRIs appear to be particularly helpful in IBS, possibly by an action on the serotonergic neurones in the gut.

5.41

Should patients with myalgic encephalomyelitis (ME) be treated for symptoms of depression?

ME is a complex condition which shares a number of symptoms with major depression (tiredness, lack of energy, low spirits, etc.). Some studies have reported a response to tricyclic antidepressants. In the absence of any specific treatment for the condition, I think it is always worth treating any prominent symptoms. Thus, if significant depressive symptoms are present, an antidepressant should be prescribed. They are often helpful. Many of the older tricyclic antidepressants have a sedative action, and it is therefore better to use the more stimulant type of antidepressants such as fluoxetine or possibly desipramine.

5.42

How should depression be treated in people with physical disabilities?

Being physically disabled can be a frustrating and depressing experience. Limited mobility, poor access to public places, sexual problems and physical discomfort probably all contribute as well. Disabled people should be asked to express how they feel. Depressive symptoms are a common concomitant of physical disability. Depression affects 36% of those with central nervous system (CNS) involvement and 20% of those with physical disability. Depression can be treated with antidepressant drugs in the usual way, but support and activity are also important. Occupational therapists may be able to advise on adaptations to the home and help with housing and mobility is important. Disabled people with sexual problems should be referred to a specialist where appropriate.

5.43

What are the signs of depression in people with learning difficulties?

Depression may be difficult to diagnose in those with learning difficulties because they are often less articulate. This group has difficulty with verbal communication, but there may be behavioural changes such as poor dress, restlessness, irritability and an alteration in personality. Sufferers may also exhibit tearfulness and a lack of normal enthusiasm for activities. Carers will be able to provide indications of depression such as not eating, poor sleeping and weight loss. Workers at day centres are also in a good position to observe depressive symptoms.

<h2>5.44</h2>

How should depressive symptoms be treated in schizophrenic patients?

Many schizophrenic patients show depressive symptoms as part of the negative pattern of symptoms which is so central to the illness – those of blunting of affect, poverty of emotional expression and general social withdrawal. These symptoms are difficult to treat at the best of times. Other patients manifest depressive symptoms as part of the abnormal mood resulting from the illness itself, or become depressed as they recover from an acute episode and realize the extent of their problem. Many patients appear to have developed depression as a secondary phenomenon to the disease process.

If the depression seems to be prodromal to a relapse, or is a symptom of undertreated psychosis, then increasing neuroleptic medication should prove helpful. Conversely, if depression is part of the Parkinsonian syndrome, or the result of sedation due to over-medication, the dosage of antipsychotic drug could be reduced, or the patient prescribed one of the newer, less sedative, more stimulating antipsychotic drugs, such as sulpiride, sertindole or olanzapine, which have lower levels of side effects. They may also be more effective against the negative symptoms of schizophrenia. In practice, many patients benefit from antidepressant medication, and a trial of an antidepressant for a few weeks may make schizophrenic patients feel better.

6 PHARMACO-THERAPY FOR ANXIETY

Introduction

Despite their efficacy in acute use, the problems associated with long-term benzodiazepine use have resulted in a re-evaluation of alternative pharmacological treatments.

6.1

How are the physical symptoms of anxiety best treated?

If patients complain of clear-cut physical symptoms such as duodenal ulcers, exacerbated by stress, the primary treatment would probably be directed at treating the ulcer, which would include measures such as H_2 blockers and advice to stop smoking. Measures to deal with underlying stress would be secondary. Equally, symptoms attributable to excessive activity of the masseter muscle, giving rise to dental problems and headaches, can be treated by using a bite guard dental prosthesis at night while waiting for the benefits of relaxation training. Patients who worry excessively about symptoms such as palpitations are best treated by reassurance and an explanation of the physical mechanisms of anxiety. For example, an explanation that palpitations are not a sign of an impending heart attack, but a normal physiological response of the heart to stress, may be valuable. When symptoms are more diffuse, and the underlying mechanism more obvious, treatments should be directed at the underlying pathology, ideally through relaxation training, reassurance and simple counselling. When panicky symptoms are severe, beta-blockers or antidepressants (Ch. 7) may be indicated.

BENZODIAZEPINES

6.2

When is it appropriate to prescribe benzodiazepines?

Benzodiazepines offer patients an effective and safe short-term treatment for severe anxiety disorders. Judicious prescribing of these powerful drugs, and adherence to the Commitee on the Safety of Medicines (CSM) recommendations (see Question 6.19), can produce beneficial results.

6.3

Why are anti-anxiety drugs licensed for the short-term treatment of anxiety when most patients end up taking them long term?

One view is that most anxiety disorders are short-lived, self-limiting conditions, and that benzodiazepines lose their therapeutic effects after a period of time as dependence develops. These patients cease to benefit from them after a few weeks' use and only continue on them because of dependency and to avoid withdrawal symptoms. Another explanation is that anxiety disorders are not the benign, short-lived conditions that they were originally thought to be when product licences were granted in the 1960s for many of the current anxiolytics. There is an increasing awareness of the chronicity of some anxiety disorders. For newer treatments under development, longer-term indications will be sought.

6.4

How do benzodiazepines work?

They act by stimulating the benzodiazepine receptor which is part of the GABA receptor complex, thus increasing GABA activity. GABA is the most widespread neurotransmitter in the CNS and has an inhibitory action.

6.5

What is the equivalent dose of the common benzodiazepines to 5 mg of diazepam?

There is no direct equivalent dosage since the drugs vary not only in potency, but in half-life, lipid solubility, metabolism and possibly intrinsic activity. However, a rough clinical equivalent is listed in Table 6.1.

Table 6.1   Approximate equivalent dose of benzodiazepines to 5 mg diazepam

Benzodiazepine	Dose
Alprazolam	0.25 mg
Chlordiazepoxide	15 mg
Loprazolam	5 mg
Lorazepam	0.5 mg
Oxazepam	15 mg
Temazepam	10 mg
Nitrazepam	5 mg

6.6

Triazolam was a very effective hypnotic drug. Can you comment on the reason it was withdrawn in Britain and suggest suitable alternatives?

Triazolam, the most potent short half-life benzodiazepine sleeping pill, was withdrawn rather suddenly because of increasing adverse reports, including rebound anxiety between doses and rebound insomnia on ending treatment. Serious paradoxical reactions such as aggression, excitation and features of psychosis, memory impairment and fatal overdose had been reported. Thus, the Committee for Proprietary Medicine Products withdrew the drug rather suddenly for legal reasons. Subsequent recommendations that the drug should be made available again have been rejected. There is no obvious substitute for triazolam, although lormetazepam at a dose of 1 to 2 mg or zopiclone at a dose of 7.5 mg at night is probably the best alternative.

6.7

What are the unwanted effects of benzodiazepines?

They commonly cause sedation during the initial phases of treatment and can give rise to hangover the following morning if taken as hypnotics. They cause psychomotor impairment, and this makes driving vehicles hazardous during the first few days of treatment.

These effects diminish with time. They also have effects upon memory which can be beneficial when used for minor operative procedures, but can also be a problem. It appears these memory effects are subtle but long-lived. In the elderly, metabolites of long-acting benzodiazepines can accumulate, resulting in chronic intoxication and acute confusional states which may simulate dementia. Benzodiazepines also potentiate alcohol and are commonly taken in combination. There are idiosyncratic reactions such as the release of aggression in certain circumstances and a host of other minor side effects. In the elderly, because of confusion and muscle relaxation, they can precipitate falls. Longer-term use results in tolerance, dependence and withdrawal reactions. Side effects are minor and rare.

6.8

Are benzodiazepines 'safe' in overdose?

Apart from a few rare instances, it is virtually impossible for someone to die from a benzodiazepine overdose. Benzodiazepines act by modulating GABA function to some degree but are not able to block the system totally. Thus, they cannot switch off the system totally as barbiturates can. However, they do potentiate alcohol and other drugs taken in overdose and are therefore hazardous in this situation.

6.9

Why is there a great disparity in the reaction to benzodiazepines?

The more anxious the patient, the greater the tolerance to benzodiazepines. Some patients can take 10 mg of diazepam or more three times a day, while others are sedated by a 2 mg dose.

Benzodiazepines reduce arousal. Highly anxious patients are over-aroused and generally seek a reduction in arousal, whereas non-anxious people become sedated if their arousal level is reduced. They are therefore more severely affected by the medication.

Tolerance develops rapidly to the sedative effects, but probably more slowly to the anxiolytic effect. In highly anxious patients who are coping badly with their symptoms there is a tendency to increase the dose as sedation wears off in the hope of achieving some relief from their highly disabling symptoms. What is interesting is why most patients do not escalate their doses and tend to stay at between 10 and 15 mg of diazepam, or equivalent, per day over long periods of time.

Dependence

6.10
How big a problem is benzodiazepine dependence?

A typical GP with a list of 2000 patients will have 60 patients taking benzodiazepines daily for a year, half of whom will have been on them for 5 years. Just over half of this group will have been taking them as night-time hypnotics, three-quarters of the patients will be over 60 years of age. About a third of these patients will be physically or psychologically dependent on the medication and will suffer withdrawal syndromes if the drug is stopped suddenly.

6.11
Why are the more effective benzodiazepines more habit-forming?

Benzodiazepines vary in their potency. For example 10 mg of diazepam is approximately equivalent to 1 mg of lorazepam and 0.125 mg of triazolam. Also, it appears that the lower the potency of the drug, the longer the half-life. Other pharmacological differences such as fat solubility and degrees of partial agonism in the receptor may be important. Thus, the more powerful drugs bind to receptors more strongly and are removed more rapidly, thereby initially giving good symptomatic relief but presumably allowing tolerance to their effects to develop more rapidly, and allowing withdrawal to be more dramatic and rapid when the drug is stopped.

6.12

Why is the problem of dependence so much worse with lorazepam than diazepam?

Lorazepam is about 10 times more potent than diazepam, locking onto the receptor more effectively. It also has a much shorter half-life. The implication is, by analogy, that of pulling a plaster off. It is much more painful to pull it off quickly if it is stuck on firmly than pulling it off slowly if the adhesive is weak. There are probably other factors related to the intrinsic activity of the drug which are ill understood.

6.13

How quickly can benzodiazepine dependency develop?

Dependency probably develops in a third of people who have taken benzodiazepines for more than 3 months, although mild rebound phenomena may be seen after a couple of weeks of sleeping pills.

6.14

What are the early warning signs of benzodiazepine dependence?

Early warning signs of dependency are hard to define, but there should be concern about the patient who continues taking benzodiazepines after about 3 or 4 weeks without there being any appreciable change in the pathological process: there would be little reason for him or her to stop taking them in the future. Drug-seeking behaviour and escalation of the dose are relatively rare, but any patient who felt unable to go for a day without benzodiazepine should give cause for worry. Dependence in itself may of course not be pathological, but represent an attempt at treating a long-term anxiety disorder.

6.15

Is there a certain type of patient who is more likely to become dependent on benzodiazepines?

Patients with a history of previous drug or alcohol dependency, or those with dependent personalities. In those with long-standing symptoms, medication will only suppress the symptoms, which will inevitably return when the medication is stopped. These patients are more likely to become dependent when offered medication. Patients with passive dependent personalities will experience more trouble discontinuing medication once they have become dependent. Patients with avoidant personalities are less likely to tolerate withdrawal symptoms and thereby will be less likely to stop medication.

6.16

Can benzodiazepine dependence be considered an addiction?

Dependency means the patient needs to continue the medication for its benefits or to avoid withdrawal symptoms. Dependency in itself is not necessarily harmful. For example, diabetics are dependent on insulin, which is to their benefit. Addiction suggests the medication is taken for non-therapeutic reasons, against medical advice, and to the detriment of the individual. The distinction between dependency and addiction is often confused.

6.17

Is benzodiazepine dependence a physical problem, or an emotional dependence?

There is no doubt that some patients will develop physical withdrawal symptoms on stopping benzodiazepines. These can include fits, psychosis, weight loss, electroencephalogram (EEG) abnormalities, muscle cramps and other diverse symptoms. Patients are also emotionally dependent on anything that makes them feel better. This in itself may not be harmful. The problem with emotional dependence is that the benzodiazepines are used to deal with the problems rather than the patient being able to confront them and deal with them in a more satisfactory way. Patients may get hooked on suppressing problems they should be dealing with. They also become psychologically reliant on the medication, needing to have it with them when they go out or they will get panics. Thus patients will have worse withdrawal problems if they have been told to expect a terrible reaction. There is obviously a strong interaction between psychological expectations and physical events. The emotions can act as triggers for physical symptoms and these in turn can have profound emotional effects.

6.18

Do patients get addicted to feeling calm and well or is there some other mechanism at work?

Patients in general get used to feeling calm and well, and possibly to a mild euphoriant effect when on benzodiazepines. Withdrawal symptoms are unrelated to feeling generally well on medication since the rebound anxiety that occurs on withdrawal can be quite dramatic and clinically distinct, both qualitatively and quantitatively, from the underlying anxiety state. It also tends to be self-limiting, although it can be difficult to distinguish between withdrawal symptoms and a recurrence of underlying anxiety symptoms. The most compelling argument in favour of the existence of dependence on benzodiazepines rather than on feeling well is that patients have little trouble stopping major tranquillizers and antidepressants, which are probably as effective as benzodiazepines in the treatment of anxiety (although they may suffer a recurrence of the underlying disorder in time). They do not suffer the dramatic withdrawal reaction and do not live their lives around getting more antidepressants.

6.19

How can we prescribe benzodiazepines and ensure our patients do not develop dependence on them?

The CSM guidelines should be adhered to. You should select patients with sound personalities, who are unlikely to abuse medication; limit prescriptions to low doses; and review prescriptions to ensure that patients do not stay on the medications for more than 2 to 3 weeks. Patients should also be encouraged to take medication as required rather than on a regular basis.

Box 6.1   CSM GUIDELINES ON PRESCRIBING BENZODIAZEPINES

1. Benzodiazepines are indicated for the short-term relief (2 to 3 weeks only) of anxiety that is severe, disabling or subjecting the individual to unacceptable distress occurring alone or in association with insomnia or short-term psychosomatic, organic or psychotic illness.
2. The use of benzodiazepines to treat short-term mild anxiety is inappropriate and unsuitable.
3. Benzodiazepines should be used to treat insomnia only when it is severe, disabling or subjecting the individual to extreme distress.

6.20

In view of the risk of dependence, is it ever justifiable to prescribe benzodiazepines?

Yes. In selected cases, they may well be a very effective short-term treatment. The CSM guidelines should be observed, patients should be advised of the risks of dependence and side effects and should be monitored appropriately. Benzodiazepines should, of course, be continued in patients who are already dependent on them and who are unable to discontinue them.

6.21

Why is the use of tranquillizers frowned upon for anxious patients in difficult social situations?

Poor housing, unemployment, alcohol abuse and non-existing nursery facilities are all common social factors which combine to make life pretty miserable. Often tranquillizers are the only thing likely to make life more bearable, especially as patients are unlikely to be able to change their circumstances or benefit much from the limited psychotherapy on offer.

One thread of the argument against benzodiazepines is that tranquillizers are handed out by the medical establishment in order to keep unhappy people relatively content, rather than complaining too much about their disadvantaged role in society. This is the political argument. The second argument is that, if benzodiazepines do work in relieving social suffering, the effects are short lived, and very soon the situation returns to the way it was before, but with the patient now dependent on the medication both physiologically and psychologically, and suffering withdrawal symptoms when medication is stopped.

The Calvinist argument is that people should sort out their own problems and not ask doctors for help and support. These are arguments and not edicts. The GP has to decide how best to help his or her patient individually.

6.22

To what extent are patients' lives made intolerable by benzodiazepine dependence?

Many patients who claim their lives have been made unbearable by benzodiazepine dependence are probably suffering from inadequately treated chronic anxiety, agoraphobia and depression. Many patients have suffered some side effects from the medication, such as cognitive impairment, and possibly a worsening of their anxiety state and agoraphobia. Benzodiazepines can also act as depressants.

6.23

If we do prescribe benzodiazepines, can we protect ourselves against legal action by patients who claim to have been made dependent on the drug?

When prescribing for a new patient you should follow the CSM guidelines. Patients should be warned of the risk of dependency and that the drug will only be prescribed for a limited period. This warning should be recorded in your notes. If you discuss the risks and benefits of the treatment with the patient there should be no grounds for legal action. Patients who have become dependent on the drug in the past are a different problem. They should be encouraged to withdraw if appropriate. If they are unable to stop, or you in your clinical view feel

111

it is inappropriate, the situation should be discussed with the patient, and the discussion recorded in the notes. If patients wish to continue taking the medication, it may be worth asking them to sign a disclaimer against future litigation. In practice, there are many patients on long-term benzodiazepines, especially sleeping pills, so the danger of litigation is receding.

Withdrawal

6.24

How troublesome are the rebound symptoms after tranquillizer withdrawal and how can they be managed?

Most patients can stop benzodiazepines without major problems. About one-third suffer some symptoms for a limited period of time which they can usually cope with. A few people suffer quite severe reactions, including withdrawal fits and psychotic episodes, but these are rare.

The management of withdrawal symptoms involves reducing the medication gradually, possibly switching to a longer-acting benzodiazepine, putting the patient in touch with a benzodiazepine self-help group, if available, and also offering anxiety management training. Some patients may need substitute medication to cover their withdrawal, either phenobarbitone (if in hospital), carbamazepine or antidepressants if they are depressed, and they should be offered self-help material either as cassettes or books. The patient should be offered support safe in the knowledge that withdrawal symptoms will subside, within a few weeks or months in most instances, after medication has been stopped. This will, of course, leave the underlying problems and anxiety states, for which the medication was prescribed, still to be addressed.

6.25

What are the common benzodiazepine withdrawal phenomena?

There are three main types of symptoms seen in tranquillizer withdrawal:

1. A rebound and increase in anxiety symptoms with panicky symptoms as well, including tension, irritability, agitation and restlessness. Some patients also become significantly depressed.
2. A group of symptoms more characteristic of benzodiazepine withdrawal, relating to a hyperstimulation of the sensory modalities. They include an intolerance of bright lights, loud noises and strong smells and possibly tinnitus.
3. A rare group of symptoms related to a delirium tremens-type syndrome in which patients can have epileptiform fits, delusions, hallucinations and perceptual distortions.

Box 6.2   COMMON BENZODIAZEPINE WITHDRAWAL SYMPTOMS

Anxiety
- Sleep disturbance
- Anxiety
- Dysphasia
- Muscular pains
- Tremor
- Shaking
- Headache
- Nausea, anorexia, weight loss
- Sweating

Distorted perception
- Visual disturbance
- Hypersensitivity to loud noise or bright lights
- Abnormal bodily sensations
- Sensations or abnormal movement
- Depersonalization

Major incident
- Psychosis
- Epileptiform seizure.

6.26

How much of a problem are epileptiform fits following benzodiazepine withdrawal?

They are relatively rare, occurring in maybe 1% of patients. They are more common when the drugs are stopped suddenly, especially if alcohol is also involved, or when a patient is admitted to hospital for intercurrent illness and the medication is stopped suddenly. The risk is reduced if the medication is withdrawn gradually. If problems are anticipated, withdrawal can be covered by either carbamazepine or phenobarbitone. Both these drugs are also useful in attenuating withdrawal symptoms. If fits occur, benzodiazepine should be reinstated immediately and withdrawn more gradually under anticonvulsant cover.

6.27

What is the GP's role in benzodiazepine withdrawal?

GPs are best placed to withdraw patients from benzodiazepines. They have an established relationship with their patients and are in a position to monitor prescriptions during withdrawal. If all long-term benzodiazepine users were referred to a specialist, the service would be overwhelmed. The most effective strategy overall is to review long-term users and advise them to phase out their medication over the next few months. This simple procedure will result in about one in five patients stopping their medication without untoward effect. This is a highly cost-effective procedure. The remainder should be offered help in reducing their medication with a reducing schedule over a 2- to 3-month period. Using a gradual, flexible withdrawal regimen and continued support, as many as half of this group should manage to withdraw without too many difficulties. The remaining patients may need to be referred to a specialist clinic, with input from clinical psychologists, etc., although with these patients the results are less satisfactory.

6.28

Is it worth switching patients on lorazepam and other benzodiazepines to diazepam before attempting to reduce the dosage?

Lorazepam and alprazolam may be the most difficult benzodiazepines to stop, and by switching to another benzodiazepine half the battle may be won. By substituting 10 mg of diazepam in 2 mg tablets for 1 mg of lorazepam, patients can appreciate how much medication they were on when they see the mountain of pills they now have to take in place of the one tiny tablet. By prescribing 2 mg tablets, it is easier to reduce the dose by 2 or 3 mg per week. Or, the Penn diazepam serial dilution pack may be used (see Question 6.29).

When taking patients off lorazepam, it is better to prescribe generous doses of diazepam to make the process easier and to encourage compliance, rather than cutting down at the same time as making the switch.

6.29

What is the Penn diazepam withdrawal kit?

This consists of two bottles, one of diazepam elixir 5 mg in 5 ml, the other of dilutent. The patient removes 5 ml of elixir as the dose and replaces it with 5 ml dilutent. Thus, the elixir becomes increasingly dilute and the patient gradually tapers off the diazepam. Hopefully, this gradual taper results in fewer withdrawal problems. Further information on the kit can be obtained from Penn Pharmaceuticals (tel: +44 (0) 1494 816 655).

6.30

Are any drugs useful during the benzodiazepine withdrawal period?

Unfortunately, there is no wonder drug to detoxify benzodiazepine users. Propanolol may be of some benefit in patients who find autonomic symptoms such as palpitations troublesome. Tricyclic antidepressants may be useful in helping sleep disturbance because of their sedative effect, and are certainly helpful in relieving depressive symptoms. As many as one-third of patients who withdraw from benzodiazepines develop significant depression. This should be treated with an appropriate antidepressant. Buspirone has no beneficial effect in benzodiazepine withdrawal and low-dose neuroleptics are of dubious benefit beyond their sedative properties. Chlormethiazole is probably effective, but is as addictive as benzodiazepines. It appears that carbamazepine and phenobarbitone, given at relatively high doses during withdrawal and continued for a couple of weeks, may be of some real value, but probably only to be prescribed for inpatients or when the patient can be monitored closely.

115

6.31

What can I do for patients who are unwilling to stop taking tranquillizers (particularly lorazepam)?

All long-term benzodiazepine users should be reviewed and offered advice and support on reduction. If patients are really unwilling to cut down medication, despite advice, then withdrawal will be difficult. You may choose to concentrate your efforts on other patients who are more willing, and review the unwilling ones at some future time; but the outcome of dealing with patients who are resistant to withdrawal is often unsatisfactory. Some patients find stopping very difficult because of severe anxiety symptoms, depression, or even outside social factors. Therapeutic failures should be offered a referral to a specialist who may advise maintaining them on the medication. About one-third of this group, even with the most experienced help, will be unable to stop their medication with the current therapies available. If a decision is taken to abandon withdrawal attempts, the decision should be recorded in the notes and patients should be offered adequate supplies of benzodiazepines to enable them to take the appropriate amount of medication. In these circumstances, they should not be prescribed a reduced dose, so that they end up with the worst of both worlds, taking benzodiazepines and still having symptoms.

6.32

What are the alternatives to benzodiazepines?

For anxiety, antidepressants, both traditional SSRIs and MAOIs, could be considered. Buspirone, beta-blockers, low doses of neuroleptics and, as hypnotics, sedative antidepressants are useful, especially if the patient is depressed. Alternatively sedative neuroleptics or chlormethiazole may be prescribed (Table 6.2).

Table 6.2 Alternative drugs for treating anxiety

Drug	Advantages	Disadvantages
Antidepressants	Effective, especially for panic and depression	Side effects may be troublesome
Beta-blockers	Good for somatic symptoms	Weak anxiolytic
Buspirone	Good anxiolytic	Slow onset of action Limited efficacy in patients who are pre-treated with benzodiazepines
Neuroleptics	Reasonable anxiolytic	Generally unpleasant to take Risk of tardive dyskinesia and Parkinsonism
Chlormethiazole	Effective anxiolytic and hypnotic	As addictive as benzodiazepines

BETA-BLOCKERS

6.33

Do beta-blockers have a place in the treatment of anxiety?

Beta-blockers appear to treat the somatic symptoms of mild anxiety and are therefore appropriate specifically for those people who complain of the somatic symptoms of anxiety and little else, for example, actors who go on the stage and find a racing heart distracting or billiards players and target shooters who find a small tremor very awkward (the use of beta-blockers is banned in competition). Musicians, such as violinists and trumpeters, perform better on beta-blockers and these drugs may be useful for examination nerves. A businessman who found blushing during business meetings distressing had his symptoms alleviated by taking propanolol. These agents are not effective in people with severe pervasive anxiety, and psychic symptoms.

6.34

What is the optimum dosage regimen of beta-blockers in the treatment of anxiety symptoms?

Patients should be encouraged to titrate the dose they need to suppress their autonomic response. It is usual to start patients on 10 mg of propanolol and teach them to monitor their pulse rates. They should then practise increasing the dose on a daily basis until they either achieve symptomatic control or 'beta-blockade', whereby their exercising pulse rate remains at about 70 beats per minute. Most patients benefit from between 40 and 80 mg of propanolol three times a day.

6.35

Is buspirone a good anxiolytic drug?

Buspirone is an effective anxiolytic if given to the right patient. It does not work for panic disorders and is not a treatment for benzodiazepine withdrawal. It also has a complex neurochemical interaction with benzodiazepines and does not work well in patients who have previously been treated with a benzodiazepine. Thus, if a patient has received a benzodiazepine in the preceding year, the therapeutic effect of buspirone is limited. Secondly, when buspirone first appeared as an alternative to benzodiazepines, many patients were switched to the new agent. This produced benzodiazepine withdrawal symptoms, and it is known that buspirone is ineffective in treating this condition. Thirdly, even where buspirone is effective, it has a gradual onset of action, in many ways similar to an antidepressant, and patients need to persevere for 3 or 4 weeks at an adequate dosage (between 20 and 30 mg daily) to get a proper therapeutic effect. This is in marked contrast to the near-instantaneous benefit seen with benzodiazepines. Finally, it has the 5-HT side-effect profile of dizziness, light-headedness, headache and nausea which some patients cannot tolerate. However, when prescribed appropriately, buspirone can be of considerable benefit, especially in general practice, for patients with relatively stable anxiety states.

6.36

Are there any other anxiolytic drugs in the pipeline?

Development of anxiolytic agents is a growth industry. There are a host of buspirone-like 5-HT$_{1A}$ agonists around, including ipsaperone and flesinoxan, which appear similar to buspirone as effective anxiolytics.

There is an increasing literature about the benefit of antidepressants for the treatment of anxiety. Most interestingly, a new reversible MAO-A (RIMA) inhibitor is available. Although this compound is to be licensed for the treatment of depression, it may have an anxiolytic action in atypical depressive states and may well be useful where other treatments fail. The benzodiazepines are still being developed. Alpidem and zolpidem are partial agonists at the benzodiazepine receptor, and these drugs appear to be as effective as benzodiazepines without some of the side effects. Other benzodiazepines with interesting pharmacological profiles are also being assessed, as are exotic compounds such as cholecystokinins.

7 PHYSICAL TREATMENTS FOR DEPRESSION

Introduction

Antidepressants should be used for moderate to
severe depression as defined by a score of greater
than 15 on the Hamilton Depression Rating Scale
(see Fig. 1.2), or if patients present with three or
more of the core symptoms – depressed mood,
pessimistic thoughts, suicidal feelings, sleep
disturbance, appetite disturbance and reduced
energy. Symptoms should be likely to persist for at
least 4 to 6 weeks to justify the time delay before the
medication works. It is the severity and persistence
of the symptoms, rather than their cause, which
should act as an indicator to initiating treatment.
ECT should be considered for severe or resistant
cases.

ANTIDEPRESSANTS

7.1

What advice should be given to patients who are starting antidepressants?

The most important information is that the drug needs as long as 3 weeks before the benefit is felt, and needs to be taken at a proper dose for the correct period of time if it is to be effective. There is little point in taking antidepressants intermittently. Patients should be told about likely side effects, such as sedation, dry mouth, constipation and possible nausea and jitteriness, depending on which medication is prescribed. They should be advised to persist in taking the medication despite side effects. If these are intolerable, the patients should come back to the GP to discuss the problem so that an alternative can be found, rather than lapsing from treatment. Patients should be assured that antidepressants, unlike benzodiazepines, are not habit-forming, and are not simply sedatives or tranquillizers.

7.2

What should I tell patients when they ask how long they should take antidepressants for?

Patients may find it helpful to know that if they get a benefit from antidepressants after taking them for 3 or 4 weeks, that there is a 50% risk of relapse in the following weeks if they stop the medication. Antidepressants are usually prescribed for a further 6 months after the patient feels well, in order to avoid a relapse. It is for the patient then to decide whether the benefits of treatment outweigh the risks of relapse.

7.3

Is any antidepressant agent more effective than any other?

Clomipramine appears to be marginally more effective than other antidepressants, but the side effects are rather hard to tolerate. Beyond that, there is little evidence for the superior effectiveness of any one antidepressant, although there are always reports of patients who have failed to respond to one antidepressant but respond to another. The exception to this appears to be MAOIs, which appear to have a different spectrum of activity, especially in the more anxious and phobic patient. They have a different mode of action and are generally underrated.

Those acting on 5-HT preferentially may be more effective in certain anxiety states than those acting on noradrenaline. In order to detect any meaningful therapeutic differences between the antidepressants, the drugs have to be tested in comparative clinical studies where patient numbers are into the hundreds. This means it is difficult for a GP, treating relatively few depressed patients with heterogenous symptoms, to be in a position to detect these differences. The therapeutic profiles of the main antidepressants are outlined in Table 7.1.

7.4

How do the side effects compare between the different antidepressant agents?

The major differences between the antidepressants are in their side-effect profiles and overdose risk. Side effects appear to be less in the newer agents (Table 7.2).

7.5

Does alcohol react with any of the common antidepressants?

Alcohol potentiates the older sedative antidepressants, resulting in significant psychomotor impairment and sedation. This does not appear to be a problem with the newer SSRIs. These drugs may even reduce the craving for alcohol in some patients.

It is important for patients to stop drinking before initiating treatment so that their depression can be assessed. If significant depressive symptoms remain, then treatment with an antidepressant is indicated, since relief of the depression will reduce the urge to drink.

Name	Approximate daily dose	Anticholinergic	Seratonergic	Noradrenergic	Sedative	Epileptogenic	Cardiotoxicity	Danger in overdose	Comment
TRICYCLICS									
Amitriptyline (Tryptizol)	150 mg	+++	++	++	+++	++		+++	The standard tricyclic
Clomipramine (Anafranil)	150 g	++	+++	+	++	++	++	++	The most effective antidepressant
Dothiepin (Prothiaden)	150 mg	++	++	++	+++	++	++	+++	The most widely prescribed in Britain
Lofepramine (Gamanil)	210 mg	+	0	++	+	+	0	0	A modern tricyclic, low on side effects
Trimipramine (Surmontil)	200 mg	++	+	+	+++	+	++	++	The most sedative tricyclic
Imipramine (Tofranil)	150 g	+++	++	+++	++	++	++	++	Another good standard, used in panic disorder
OTHERS									
Mianserin (Bolvidon/Norval)	60 mg	0	++	0	+++	0	0	0	Atypical antidepressant. Less side effects. Sedative, safe in elderly Rare blood dyscrasias
Nefazodone (Dutonin)	400 mg	0	+++	0	0	+	0	?	Blocks 5-HT2 receptors as well as SSRI effects
Trazodene (Molipaxin)	200 mg	0	+++	0	++	+	+	+	A sedative antidepressant

Table 7.1   Therapeutic profiles of some antidepressants

Drug	Dose				Stimulant			Comments
SSRIs								
Fluoxetine (Prozac)	20 mg	0	+++	0	+	0	0	Different/better side effect profile than traditional tricyclic antidepressants
Fluvoxamine (Faverin)	150 mg	0	+++	0	+	0	0	
Sertrazine (Lustral)	100 mg	0	+++	0	+	0	0	
Paroxitine (Seroxat)	20 mg	0	+++	0	+	0	0	
Citalopram (Cipramil)	40 mg	0	+++	0	?	0	0	The most potent SSRI
SNRIs								
Venlafaxine (Effexor)	150 mg	0	+++	0	?	0	?	4th generation antidepressants. Tricyclic profile without side effects
Mirtazapine (Zispin)	30 mg	+	+++	++	?	0	0	Complex actions. Lacks SSRIs side effects
NARI								
Reboxitine (Edronax)	8 mg	0	0	0	?	0	?	Selective noradrenergic reuptake inhibitor. Different mode of action
MAOIs								
Phenelzine (Nardil)	45–90 mg in daily divided doses	–	++	0	–	0	++	Safest MAOI. Least stimulant
Isocarboxazid (Marplan)	as for Phenelzine	–	++	0	–	0	++	As for Phenelzine
Tranylcypromine (Parnate)	10–30 mg, given before noon	–	++	0	–	0	++	Stimulant with amphetamine-like effects
Moclebamide (Manerix)	300–600 mg, to be taken after meals	–	++	++	–	0	0	A RIMA

Table 7.2 Main differences in side effects of older TCAs and SSRIs

Older TCAs (mostly common and mild)	SSRIs (rare but may be intolerable)
Dry mouth	Nausea
Constipation	Vomiting
Hypotension	Headache
Sedation	Sexual difficulties
Weight gain	
Cardiac toxicity	
Danger in overdose	

Prescribing antidepressants in someone who continues to drink excessively is a hazardous procedure. Modest amounts of alcohol are probably safe in conjunction with the SSRIs.

7.6

Is there a safe, effective antidepressant that can be used in pregnancy?

It is best to avoid all medication during pregnancy, and fortunately depression is relatively rare during pregnancy. Giving medication in the third trimester is less hazardous than in the second trimester, and it is probably best to use imipramine or amitriptyline since there is the most experience with these drugs to date. Ultimately, it is necessary to balance the risk of harm to the fetus from treatment against benefits to the mother. The individual risk is small but can be catastrophic if birth defects arise. Most prospective mothers will choose to avoid taking antidepressants during pregnancy. Consider psychotherapeutic alternatives.

7.7

Is there an antidepressant which can be used in the puerperium if the mother is breast-feeding?

The well-tried standards of imipramine or amitriptyline are probably treatments of choice. If the mother is so depressed as to require medication, she will probably not want to breast-feed. If she is breast-feeding, these drugs are excreted in very small amounts in the breast milk, and although detectable amounts will be found in the baby, especially when it is young, these are probably relatively safe.

7.8

Do patients become dependent on antidepressants in the same way that they become dependent on benzodiazepines?

No. Benzodiazepine dependence is regarded as pathological because of the lack of evidence of long-term efficacy and because of the phenomenon of a marked rebound withdrawal syndrome in some patients when the medication is stopped. There is associated craving and some people have great difficulty discontinuing medication. With tricyclics, there is generally no problem in stopping treatment. The main problem is keeping patients on the medication for long enough. On abrupt discontinuation some patients experience transient mild symptoms which are thought to result from the withdrawal of the anticholinergic effect. Other patients complain of anxiety and sleep disturbance with vivid dreaming, and a few cases of over-activity have been described. These are unlike the symptoms of depression, and of a milder degree, and are overcome by a gradual reduction of dosage. Patients do relapse if medication is stopped, but this usually occurs some time after the medication is withdrawn and is seen as a return of the underlying illness rather than a withdrawal effect of the medication. The situation with MAOIs is somewhat different, especially tranylcypromine which has an amphetamine-like action. Tolerance to the effects occurs in time, and the dose may need to be increased. Patients can become quite dysphoric on discontinuing the medication and become psychologically dependent on its beneficial effects. With all medication that is perceptibly beneficial, patients are wary of stopping taking it and are to some degree psychologically dependent.

7.9

Should antidepressants be discontinued suddenly, or should they be reduced in dosage and tailed off gently?

It is good practice to discontinue all medication gradually. This is more important with the sedative anticholinergic antidepressants with relatively short half-lives such as desipramine. In such cases, cholinergic rebound and release from sedation may give rise to transient symptoms. The medication should be tailed off over a week or two. Compounds without anticholinergic or sedative properties and with long half-lives, such as fluoxetine, can be stopped abruptly without untoward effects. Paroxitime needs to be tailed off.

TRICYCLICS

7.10

How do tricyclic antidepressants work in the treatment of depression?

Tricyclic antidepressants act by blocking the reuptake of the neurotransmitters, 5-HT, dopamine and noradrenaline from the synaptic cleft, thereby increasing their concentrations and thus their ability to stimulate post-synaptic receptors. This theory has the advantage of explaining some of the phenomena we observe, but is insufficient to explain the entire situation. For example, this effect occurs within minutes or hours, although it takes 3 weeks for a full therapeutic effect. Thus, other mechanisms must also be important. It appears that down-regulation of post-synaptic receptors also takes place, and presumably secondary transmitter systems are also involved (Fig. 7.1). Although we know a great deal about the effects of these drugs, we are a long way short of the full story.

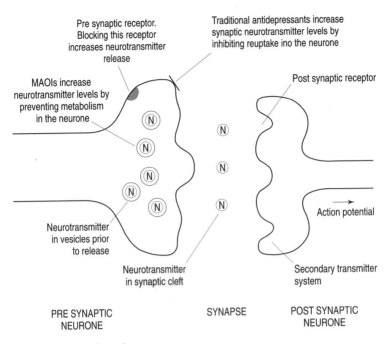

Fig. 7.1 Sites of antidepressant action.

7.11

What is the most widely prescribed drug from this group?

Prothiaden is the market leader in the UK. The reason for this is primarily historical since it was the first second-generation antidepressant to be introduced, in 1969. It has maintained its position ever since. Interestingly, other European countries have their own particular favourites, some of which are hardly prescribed at all in the UK. For example, viloxazine is very popular in the Benelux countries, and virtually unused in the UK. These are primarily aspects of marketing.

7.12

What sort of antidepressant drug is lofepramine?

Lofepramine is a tricyclic antidepressant. It is extensively metabolized to desipramine, but is an active antidepressant in its own right. It has the advantage of being low in cardiotoxicity and relatively devoid of anticholinergic and sedative side effects. It is one of the safer drugs from the point of view of overdose, appears to have distinct advantages over the traditional older tricyclics and stands up well against the modern SSRIs.

7.13

How does lofepramine differ from the older tricyclics?

There is very little difference apart from the absence of a free NH_2 group in the side-chain, which makes it relatively devoid of anticholinergic side effects. On the other hand, after repeated dosage, significant amounts of desipramine, a metabolite of imipramine, are present in the blood.

7.14

How effective is lofepramine?

It appears to be as effective as the older tricyclics with a much improved profile of side effects and is relatively well tolerated by patients. It would therefore appear to be a good antidepressant. The dose is one tablet 2 to 3 times a day (140 to 210 mg daily).

7.15

How safe is lofepramine taken as an overdose?

Lofepramine appears much safer than other tricyclic antidepressants when taken in overdose. Figures from the first 1.5 million prescriptions show there has been no death from overdose alone, and only two in combination with other drugs. It appears that lofepramine may even prevent the harmful effects of desipramine on the heart.

7.16

What is the therapeutic dosage of tricyclic antidepressants?

This is an area where GPs and psychiatrists tend to disagree. In general doses of above 125 mg of amitriptyline, imipramine or dothiepin should be within the therapeutic range. If that fails, it may be necessary to increase the dosage. In the US, it is not unusual to give doses of up to 300 mg of imipramine. In general practice, much lower doses, such as dothiepine 25 mg at night, are frequently prescribed, and GPs claim therapeutic successes. Unfortunately, studies in general practice patients have consistently shown that 75 mg of a tricyclic antidepressant is no better than placebo, although patients in this group have quite a high placebo response. These drugs also have sedative qualities, which may be interpreted as of therapeutic benefit in some patients. If dosage represents a problem, plasma levels can be measured to see if they fall within an effective range or therapeutic window.

7.17

Is it necessary to titrate upwards with the newer antidepressants?

The newer antidepressants can be started at the full therapeutic dose, without having to titrate upwards. It is still possible to increase the dose two- or threefold if there is lack of response after 3 weeks. The reason for titrating the dose up for SSRIs would be to avoid panicky feelings and other transient side effects which sometimes occur when starting on an antidepressant. If this is a problem, it may be helpful to prescribe 2 or 3 days of benzodiazepines to tide the patient over the first days of treatment.

7.18

What are the main adverse effects of the tricyclic antidepressants?

These can be mainly understood in terms of the effects of the drug on other receptor systems apart from 5-HT, dopamine and noradrenaline.

The antihistamine effects give rise to sedation and psychomotor impairment. The antihistamine action also potentiates the sedative effects of alcohol. The anticholinergic gives dry mouth, constipation, urinary retention in the elderly, glaucoma in predisposed individuals and memory problems. Alpha-blocking effects can cause postural hypotension and a quinidine-like action gives rise to cardiac conduction defects. Stimulation of noradrenergic systems can give rise to cardiac arrhythmias. Beyond that are idiosyncratic reactions such as skin rashes or hepatotoxicity, which are common to almost all medications. In some rare instances antidepressants may precipitate episodes of hypomania. Despite the daunting list of potential side effects, they are for the most part mild, wane after the first few days of treatment, and are generally tolerable, especially if the patient is warned about them and the dose increased gradually.

7.19

Which of these adverse effects are potentially serious?

Urinary retention in elderly men and glaucoma are important. Cardiac arrhythmias can in rare instances cause sudden death, although the risk of arrhythmias is only a major problem in overdose. It has to be borne in mind that in the UK approximately one person per day dies as a result of a tricyclic overdose.

7.20

Are there certain groups of patients who should not receive tricyclic antidepressants, at least not in the first instance?

The question as to whether the older tricyclic antidepressants, or the newer SSRIs (and lofepramine, a modern tricyclic antidepressant), should be used as a treatment of first choice remains uncertain. However, there are groups of patients for whom the risk of complications with the older tricyclics makes the newer drugs the treatment of first choice. Thus, in patients over 65, those at higher risk of suicide, patients with heart conditions, and those in whom major tricyclic side effects limit compliance, tricyclics should not be prescribed as first-line treatments.

7.21

Should patients continue with tricyclic antidepressants indefinitely?

It is always good to reassess patients in the light of current thinking and practice. Their notes should be reviewed carefully, especially if they were placed on long-term antidepressants by another clinician. This information and the criteria outlined in this section, together with clinical judgement in discussion with the patient's wishes, should decide any future action. However, there is a significant risk of relapse if antidepressants are stopped even after 5 years and probably longer.

7.22

In patients with marked sleep disturbance, should a hypnotic be prescribed as well as an antidepressant?

The sedative properties of some of the older antidepressant drugs – amitriptyline, dothiepin or trimipramine – are often quite useful in the treatment of depressed patients with marked sleep disturbance, or of agitated patients, with the benefit of treating these symptoms immediately while the antidepressant effect emerges over time. This has the advantage of using one drug to cover multiple symptoms. It has the disadvantage that the antihistamine sedation is often quite unpleasant, giving a heavy tired feeling rather than an anxiolytic one. Often the sedative effect is noted at quite a low dose, but it becomes difficult to increase the dose to a therapeutic level which, in the case of trimipramine, is between 150 and 300 mg. Thus, the patient may end up being sedated without the depression being treated. Newer antidepressants which are still sedative without the anticholinergic action are mianserin and trazodone. These have a different side effect profile to older antidepressants but are not without their own problems. Another option would be to give a newer antidepressant without marked sedative qualities and offer a few days' treatment with a benzodiazepine. The danger with this strategy is that patients may take the benzodiazepines and not the antidepressants and come back a week later asking for more benzodiazepines.

MIANSERIN

7.23

What class of antidepressant drug is mianserin and how does it work?

Mianserin could be regarded as a second-generation tetracyclic antidepressant with a novel mode of action. It antagonizes presynaptic alpha-2 receptors, increasing noradrenaline production, and enhances 5-HT receptor functioning. It has no anticholinergic action and is therefore beneficial for those with glaucoma and prostatism, and is quite sedative, which may be an advantage in agitated insomniac patients. It is safe in overdose.

7.24

What are the side effects of mianserin?

The most notable side effect is blood dyscrasia, which occurs in about one in 8000 prescriptions. The risk appears to be a function of dose and age, and caution should be observed in patients over 65, when the risk of agranulocytosis has to be weighed against the benefits of the lack of anticholinergic action. Blood counts should be performed every 4 weeks for the first 3 months of treatment and the drug should be withdrawn if fever develops. It is also quite sedative.

Monoamine oxidase inhibitors (MAOIs) and reversible inhibitors of monoamine oxidase A (RIMAs)

7.25

How do MAOIs work in the treatment of depression?

They act by increasing 5-HT, dopamine and noradrenaline concentrations in the synaptic cleft, but, in contrast to the reuptake inhibitors, they block the enzyme that inactivates the neurotransmitters. They may also have more complex actions, and tranylcypromine (Parnate) may also have a mild amphetamine-like action of its own.

7.26

How effective are MAOIs?

As antidepressants they are probably less effective than standard tricyclics. They appear to be particularly suitable for some patients who do not respond adequately to first-line treatments, and those with 'atypical depression', those with marked phobias or anxiety and panic attacks. In these patients they are often quite dramatically effective. They are sometimes taken for years, but in some people they lose efficacy with time.

RIMAs, the new generation of MAOIs, appear to be as effective as traditional antidepressants in major depression.

7.27

What are the rules for starting and stopping MAOIs, especially if a change to or from tricyclics is proposed?

When starting MAOIs, it is always good to start with the lowest dose tablet daily for a couple of days before increasing to the full therapeutic dose over the week. Some, such as phenelzine, are stimulant, and a usual dose is two 15 mg tablets in the morning, one or more at lunch-time, but rarely in the evening. Some people feel sedated and take the total dose in the evening. The main problem in initiating therapy is that some patients will develop postural hypotension, and this is the most troublesome side effect. Patients should be warned about it, but should be asked to tolerate it if possible. Basically, they get dizzy when they stand up. Obviously, they should be warned about dietary restrictions. If an MAOI is stopped, the patient should continue to observe the dietary restrictions for a period of 10 days.

It is highly dangerous to add a tricyclic to an MAOI, even if the MAOI was stopped within a few days: a 2-week gap must be left. Adding an antidepressant, especially clomipramine or other 5-HT reuptake inhibitors, is quite likely to prove fatal. Fluoxetine has a very long half-life, and the patient needs to be off it for 5 weeks before starting an MAOI. On the other hand, adding an MAOI to a non-5-HT reuptake inhibiting antidepressant is not hazardous and may well be therapeutic. For example, adding phenelzine to dothiepin or trimipramine is a recognized treatment. Changing from one MAOI to another can give rise to strange reactions, and it is advisable to leave a week's gap between the two. Juggling with MAOIs can be hazardous and is best left in experienced hands.

7.28

Should patients be started on MAOIs by a GP or should they be prescribed by a psychiatrist initially?

These drugs are regarded with suspicion because of the rare but fatal 'cheese reaction'. Because of this they really should be used by doctors who are used to using MAOIs. It is especially important to warn patients of the dietary restrictions. Despite the drawbacks, MAOIs are particularly effective treatments for chronic neurosis, and patients may be missing out on appropriate treatment if these drugs are not prescribed. Fortunately, new MAOIs (RIMAs) are available which show promise of providing interesting and novel therapeutic options.

7.29

What are the specific food restrictions which should be adhered to by a patient on MAOIs?

The compound to be avoided is tyramine, an amino acid resulting from the breakdown of protein. Thus, patients should avoid anything with decomposed protein. This includes cheese (which is fermented milk), pickled herrings, yeast extracts such as Marmite and fermented meat extracts such as Oxo and Bovril. Game which has been hung to enhance its flavour will have started to decompose, and some exotic continental-type sausages taste best when ripened, which requires a degree of decomposition.

Banana skins contain 5-HT, and patients should be aware of any other sympathomimetics such as ephedrine which are available in over-the-counter cough remedies. Rich red wines contain tyramine. Fresh red meat, fresh dairy produce, and ordinary gravy without meat or yeast extracts are safe, as is one glass of light white wine (Table 7.3).

Table 7.3   Foods (rich in tyramine) to avoid when taking MAOIs*

Cheese
Pickled herrings
Broad bean pods
Bovril, Oxo, Marmite (or similar meat or yeast extract), Twiglets
Alcohol (especially mature red wine); one glass of white wine is allowed daily

* Take no medicines or over-the-counter preparations without telling your doctor or pharmacist you are taking MAOIs

7.30

What should I do about a patient on MAOIs who claims to have just drunk a glass of Chianti?

In all likelihood there will be no problem. The vast number of patients do not obey the dietary restrictions to the letter and get away without a reaction. The tyramine reaction is very rare. However, a patient who consumes a tyranime-rich substance should have his or her blood pressure taken as a matter of urgency, because the tell-tale signs of impending trouble are an increase in blood pressure, headaches and a rise in body temperature.

7.31

What is a RIMA?

This is a reversible inhibitor of MAO-A. Moclobemide has recently been launched in the UK, and others may be available shortly. These are selective and reversible MAOIs and thus cause less potentiation of tyramine and are for the most part free of the risk of a cheese reaction. They appear to be an exciting new therapeutic tool, but their true therapeutic potential and safety profile need to be fully established.

SELECTIVE SEROTONIN REUPTAKE INHIBITORS (SSRIs)

7.32

How do the SSRIs affect mood?

The most widely implicated neurotransmitter in the causation or mechanism of depressive illnesses is serotonin or 5-HT. These new drugs selectively block 5-HT uptake without blocking noradrenaline, dopamine or any of the other neurotransmitters. It seems this is sufficient to give a satisfactory antidepressant, and possibly anti-anxiety, response. The new drugs have been named selective serotonin reuptake inhibitors to differentiate them from older agents. It is not so much the blocking of 5-HT that is important, but the fact that they do not block all the other neurotransmitters, which tends to avoid side effects. Their highly selective 5-HT-blocking action may possibly be important in their therapeutic effect, but this remains to be proven. Some antidepressants, such as maprotiline and lofepramine, selectively block noradrenaline and appear not to be effective in panic states.

7.33

Is there any difference in the effectiveness of the newer drugs fluoxetine, paroxetine, fluvoxamine, citalopram or sertraline?

Basically, they are similar drugs that differ in their specificity for 5-HT and, marginally, in their side-effect profiles. Fluoxetine is sometimes stimulating and may cause less weight gain than the others, especially at high doses. I think the differences are marginal.

7.34

Can SSRIs be used to treat all degrees of depression?

There is a false view that SSRIs are less potent antidepressants than the older tricyclics. They are as effective as traditional tricyclic antidepressants, with the possible exception of clomipramine which may be more effective. This, however, is of marginal significance in general practice.

7.35

When do you recommend patients should take their single dose of the SSRI, in the morning or at night?

I would suggest taking their dose nightly. Fluoxetine can be taken in the morning since it is mildly stimulant. Patients should take fluoxetine with food to reduce the incidence of nausea. Ultimately, it is a matter of patient preference and compliance as to when they choose to take the medication.

7.36

What are the commonly experienced side effects of the SSRIs?

Headache and nausea are the two characteristic SSRI side effects which occur to some degree in between 10 and 20% of patients taking them. They are, for the most part, mild. Weight gain may occur. Some patients complain of tiredness and others of insomnia (fluoxetine is especially stimulating). Sweating and dizziness, constipation and diarrhoea have also been reported, and nervousness may be a problem early in treatment when occasional panicky feelings or feeling 'hyper' have been reported. Other side effects are reported as frequently as with placebo.

7.37

Do SSRIs justify their greater expense?

It appears from the sales figures of the SSRIs that, whatever the protestations, the GPs who prescribe them and pass the costs on to third parties increasingly think that the costs are justified.

There is also interesting data on the costs of treating depression with either an SSRI or a traditional tricyclic antidepressant. If the overall costs are examined, not only of the initial prescription, but of factors such as repeat visits to the doctor if the patient experiences intolerable side effects, treating a patient who has taken an overdose, ECT treatment if the patient fails to respond to medication because of a lack

139

of tolerance to the drug, and referral to a specialist because of poor compliance, it can be shown that SSRIs are no more expensive than the older tricyclics. Psychotropic drugs in general are very cheap because they have been around so long, and are out of patent. Any new psychotropic agent is therefore seen as comparatively expensive.

When calculating drug costs, apart from companies charging what the market will bear, companies also have only a limited time to recoup their massive development costs, which are well over £100 million per drug which comes to market. Part of the cost is caused by increasing requirements for safety data, and the costs of each successful compound have to repay the thousands of unsuccessful compounds that are also undergoing development. Treatment to my mind is cheap if it works and expensive if it does not work, whatever the cost. It is clearly a complicated question, and laden with value judgements. Ultimately, it depends on who is paying the price and who is making the decision.

7.38

If the newer antidepressants are safer in overdose, can the use of the older tricyclic drugs be justified?

Despite their dramatic impact, overdoses are relatively rare occurrences in most depressed patients being treated with antidepressants. The prevention of overdosing should not be the determining factor in treating depressed patients but the effective relief of depression. Familiarity with the efficacy and side effects of a compound is an important consideration when deciding which drug to prescribe. The 'Zelmid spectre' provides a cautionary tale. Zimeledine was a very good SSRI antidepressant which was launched in the early 1980s. Unfortunately, some rare and unexpected side effects emerged only after considerable use. It is worth being slightly careful in prescribing the newest and the best immediately. However, the new SSRIs have been tested extensively, without untoward reactions.

7.39

Can a doctor be found negligent if a patient taking a tricyclic instead of an SSRI dies from an overdose?

In the UK a doctor does not have to offer the best treatment, only proper treatment. Negligence can only be established if a doctor is not matching up to standards set by a reputable body of medical opinion. Thus, if a reputable body of GPs prescribe tricyclic antidepressants to their patients, a GP cannot be found negligent in prescribing them, providing proper care has been exercised in establishing suicidal risk, and so on.

OTHER ANTIDEPRESSANTS

7.40

What is an SNRI?

This is a new class of antidepressant now available. It may be regarded as a fourth-generation antidepressant, having complex actions. Whereas the SSRIs were highly specific on 5-HT-reuptake inhibition, these new compounds have actions on more than one transmitter system whilst avoiding affecting the other less desirable neurotransmitter systems. For example, venlafaxine is a highly specific reuptake inhibitor of serotonin and noradrenaline, having a dual mode of action, much like the traditional tricyclic antidepressants, without affecting the other transmitter systems which are associated with side effects.

7.41

Is an SNRI simply a cleaner tricyclic antidepressant?

Firstly, the chemical structure is not that of any other antidepressants, and certainly not tricyclic. Secondly, its pharmacological action is also more complex so far as it down-regulates beta receptors acutely. All antidepressants are thought to down-regulate these receptors after chronic use, but this occurs after a single dose with venlafaxine, which may be a clue to its more rapid onset of action at higher doses.

141

7.42

Do we really need all these new antidepressants?

Yes. Novel modes of action provide a hope that we can treat patients
with these compounds who may hitherto have been resistant to
existing therapies. There is always a patient who will respond to one
compound and not another. Added to this of course, these new
compounds are a great deal more palatable and better tolerated than
the existing ones. Increasing activity in this therapeutic area stimulates
a more positive approach to treatment.

7.43

Are there any other antidepressants?

Nefazodone acts by 5-HT-reuptake inhibition as well as on 5-HT$_{1A}$
receptor blockade. This may reduce some of the SSRI side effects. It also
has a unique effect on restoring natural sleep patterns. Then, venlafaxine
has a dual mode of action on noradrenaline and 5-HT, but a more rapid
onset of action at higher doses. It does not have the side-effect problems
of tricyclic antidepressants. Mirtazapine has a dual mode of action
enhancing noradrenergic transmission and 5-HT$_1$ transmission.

7.44

Should flupenthixol be used in the treatment of some anxiety disorders, since it is only licensed for short-term use in mild-to-moderate depression with or without anxiety?

Most drugs are used for conditions for which they are not licensed, a
reflection of the narrow legal submission for licensing. Drugs may be
used for non-licensed indications, although it potentially lays a doctor
open to litigation if things go wrong. For example, most anxiolytics are
licensed for short-term use only but are prescribed long term, although
this is being reviewed in the case of newer anxiolytics. Flupenthixol at
a low dose of 0.5 mg twice daily works rapidly, has few acute side
effects, and is often effective when other treatments fail. This is a
general property of low-dose neuroleptics. The risk of long-term
treatment is that a proportion of patients will develop parkinsonism

and possibly tardive dyskinesia, or, most importantly, a form of akathesia marked by restlessness and anxiety (which rapidly responds to a reduction in the medication).

7.45

What are the uses of carbamazepine in psychiatry?

Carbamazepine is a tricyclic compound, a derivative of imipramine, which is primarily used in the treatment of temporal lobe epilepsy. It became evident that it also has psychotropic effects, including an improvement in mood, reduced aggressiveness and generally improved cognitive functioning. Although not licensed for these indications, it is used as a second-line prophylactic treatment for patients with bipolar mood disorders, especially in those where lithium is contraindicated. It may be of particular benefit in patients who have rapid cycling (rapid mood swings from mania to depression over a few days). It is also useful in trigeminal neuralgia and may be helpful as an adjunct to benzodiazepine withdrawal. It is useful as an adjunctive treatment, together with neuroleptics, in the treatment of resistant cases of schizophrenia, and with antidepressants for resistant depression, and is a treatment for acute mania.

While at first sight it might appear to be a universal panacea in psychiatry, the evidence for its efficacy is slight in comparison with other treatments, and it has a high incidence of skin reactions, including the dangerous Stevens–Johnson syndrome. It remains a useful second-line treatment.

7.46

Is the efficacy of carbamazepine in the treatment of trigeminal neuralgia related to the psychotropic/antidepressant effects?

No. Trigeminal neuralgia is a neurological disorder which can also be treated neurosurgically. Carbamazepine is a weak antidepressant (if it is an antidepressant at all), and only an adjunctive treatment in pain states. The mechanism of action of carbamazepine is complex, but it acts preferentially in the limbic system in the brain and has actions on many neurotransmitters. Its action is specific in trigeminal neuralgia, and not secondary to its other psychotropic effects.

7.47

Do the benzodiazepines have any real antidepressant properties?

Most benzodiazepine effects on depression are as a direct consequence of their action on the associated anxiety symptoms. Alprazolam is claimed to have antidepressant effects on the core symptoms of depression, and, while this may be true, they are not sufficient to justify its use as an antidepressant. The drug is also addictive and the treatment of depression may need to be continued long term. The inappropriate use of benzodiazepines to treat depression in the past, in the mistaken belief that they were safer than antidepressants, has in my view resulted in considerable chronic depression and unnecessary benzodiazepine dependence (see Ch. 6).

7.48

What is the next therapeutic step if an antidepressant agent is not effective?

If there has been no satisfactory response to the first-line antidepressant at full doses after 4 to 6 weeks, the next step would be to increase the dose. In the case of an SSRI this is done by doubling the dose, or, with a tricyclic, increasing it to the limit of tolerability. If this strategy fails after a further 2 weeks, it would be advisable to change to a different type of antidepressant, that is to say from an SSRI to a tricyclic or vice versa. If this fails, folic acid 5 mg should be added three times a day, which theoretically improves efficacy and appears to be harmless. Either carbamazepine or lithium could be added to the antidepressant to a level that achieves a proper therapeutic plasma concentration. After this, the diagnosis should be reconsidered. If it is still felt that the patient is significantly depressed, an MAOI could be substituted. If these all fail, ECT should be considered.

7.49

Are the newer SNRIs and NaSSAs (noradrenergic and specific serotonergic antidepressants) any better than the SSRIs?

This remains to be seen. The new compounds seem to have an even more favourable side-effect profile than the standard SSRIs and theoretically might prove more effective, although this has yet to be shown. Again what remains to be seen is whether the advantages are real or illusary. Preliminary clinical experience seems to suggest that Venlafaxine at high doses really is more effective than other antidepressants, but only time will tell. Unfortunately the better and safer antidepressants get more patients worried about side effects. This is a somewhat paradoxical response. The side-effect profiles of some of the new antidepressants are really very similar to placebo.

ELECTROCONVULSIVE THERAPY (ECT)

7.50

How does ECT work?

ECT down-regulates beta-receptors and enhances central neurotransmission in a manner similar to antidepressants. It also affects GABA-B receptors and central muscarinic receptors, which may be the mechanism of the post-therapy memory deficits. The precise mode of action remains a matter of conjecture.

7.51

What are the main indications for ECT?

ECT is primarily used for the treatment of severe depression which is not responsive to antidepressants. It is also used for patients who are in depressive stupors and unable to eat and drink, and is particularly beneficial in patients with depressive delusions. It can also be used in acute mania and psychosis. It is the most effective treatment for severe depression, and probably the safest, and is generally under-used.

7.52

Is ECT more effective in certain types of depression?

The superiority of ECT over antidepressants is most pronounced in the severely ill patient, and it is mainly kept in reserve as a treatment of

145

last resort. In the milder cases the benefit is less marked, and treatment with antidepressants is probably more acceptable.

7.53

What are the pros and cons of unilateral versus bilateral ECT?

Bilateral ECT may be more effective. Unilateral ECT given to the non-dominant hemisphere appears to cause fewer memory problems.

7.54

What are the common side effects of ECT?

The most troublesome side effect is memory loss. Patients complain of strange gaps in their memory, especially for people's names and details of events. It is maximal around the time of treatment and improves over the following weeks and months. This troublesome side effect is not universal, and needs to be balanced against the harmful effects of severe, untreated depression and prolonged hospitalization. Side effects can be minimized by giving unilateral ECT to the non-dominant hemisphere.

Otherwise, side effects are rare and limited mainly to the hazard of anaesthetic or to musculoskeletal problems, both of which are extremely rare.

7.55

Is there a limit to the total number of ECTs that can be given in a depressive illness or in a lifetime?

No. Most patients require between 6 and 10 treatments in one course. There would need to be some perceptible evidence of response before exceeding 20 treatments. There are patients who have had several hundred ECTs over a lifetime, apparently with benefit and without obvious harm.

8 LITHIUM PROPHYLAXIS

Introduction

Depression is by nature a recurrent illness associated with prolonged remission. 50% of patients suffer a relapse if medication is stopped immediately on recovery, whereas only 20% relapse over 6 months if medication is continued. After the acute episode, there is a significant risk for further episodes of depression, occurring on average every 5 years, although the frequency of recurrences increases with age. Thus, the majority of patients with established depressive illnesses suffer recurrences, although there may be prolonged periods of health in between. A phenomenon called kindling has been postulated whereby each depressive episode makes it more likely that the patient will suffer further episodes in the future. If this is true, then the prevention of relapse becomes more important.

8.1

What is the treatment of choice for prevention of relapse of long-term depressive illnesses?

The obvious choices lie between antidepressant medication and lithium. Both treatments have advantages and disadvantages (Table 8.1).

Table 8.1   Advantages and disadvantages of antidepressants compared with lithium in long-term prophylaxis

Drug	Advantages	Disadvantages
Antidepressants	Continuing established treatment for depression	Side effects. Cost of new drugs
	Ease of treatment	Bad for bipolar patients
Lithium	Established efficacy	Side effects. Regular blood tests
	Good for bipolar patients	May cause hypothyroidism
	Antidepressants can be added if the patient becomes depressed	May cause polyuria and polydipsia, but is no longer felt to be nephrotoxic

8.2

How does lithium work?

Lithium competes with sodium and other ions, thereby affecting the excitability of neuronal membranes. It also affects the metabolism of biogenic amines and has an effect on dopamine receptor sensitivity. As with antidepressants, it also affects the down-regulation of beta-adrenoreceptors. Thus, lithium has many actions, but which ones are important for its therapeutic effect remains uncertain.

8.3

What are the main indications for prescribing lithium?

Lithium is the treatment of choice in the prophylaxis of recurrent bipolar mood disorders. As a rule of thumb, if a patient has two episodes in 2 years, or three episodes in 5 years, long-term prophylaxis should be considered. In general, these phases recur more frequently in time rather than less frequently. The benefits and disadvantages of treatment should be negotiated with the patient. Lithium is also an effective treatment in acute mania, and has a useful therapeutic role in the prevention of recurrent depressive illness. It is also used as an adjunctive treatment for resistant depression and psychosis in combination with antidepressants and antipsychotics. It is sometimes used in people with difficult and aggressive personality disorders, when it occasionally has a dramatically beneficial effect on behaviour, presumably because their difficulties are amplified by minor mood fluctuations.

8.4

How effective is it in the treatment of bipolar disorder?

Lithium is the treatment of choice in the prevention of bipolar disorder, but its efficacy is unpredictable. Basically, bipolar mood disorders have a tendency to get worse over time, and treatment with lithium may only reduce the frequency or lessen the severity of the mood swings, rather than abolish them. It is hard to predict what the course of the illness would have been if the individual patient had not been prescribed lithium. In general, lithium stabilizes most patients effectively.

8.5

How soon can a patient with bipolar disorder expect to benefit from lithium therapy?

There is often a considerable time gap between starting lithium treatment and the onset of its full therapeutic benefit. Having taken the decision to initiate treatment, it is worth persisting for 2 years before evaluating its long-term efficacy in the individual.

8.6

How should patients take their daily dose of lithium?

Spacing out the medication, which results in less fluctuation of the plasma concentration and therefore in possibly fewer side effects, makes compliance more difficult. Some preparations (Priadel and Camcolit 400) are sustained-release preparations which, to some degree, overcome this problem. Once-daily dosage is probably adequate.

8.7

What is the ideal plasma concentration for lithium?

Efficacy generally increases with increasing plasma concentration, as do side effects and toxicity. In general, patients should be maintained at between 0.5 and 0.8 mmol/l, although some patients may require up to 1.2 mmol/l and some can be adequately maintained on less. Toxicity occurs above 2 mmol/l. A normal therapeutic dose of Priadel is often between 800 and 1200 mg/day.

8.8

How frequently should lithium levels be monitored?

When starting lithium, levels should be determined weekly at first, and when the desired plasma concentration and steady state have been reached, estimations can be performed monthly for a couple of months and then 3-monthly thereafter. Lithium concentrations should be determined 'in the trough', which means approximately 12 hours after the last dose, which would be the morning if the drug was taken the night before, omitting the morning dose.

8.9

Is it possible to measure saliva levels of lithium?

The ratio between salivary and plasma lithium concentrations is a
constant for the individual. Salivary lithium concentrations are usually
a little higher than plasma levels. Once the ratio has been established
by three estimations of each at different concentrations, patients may
produce a saliva specimen for regular monitoring. The specimen could
even be sent by post. This is particularly useful for patients who do not
like blood tests.

8.10

What are the main adverse effects of lithium?

Many patients experience polyuria and polydipsia. This is reversible.
Fears that lithium could cause more serious kidney damage are
probably unfounded. Patients may experience weight gain and a fine
tremor, and the most troublesome complaint is often one of a mild
lowering of mood, so that patients do not experience the pleasures of
mild highs. They also complain of a general lack of spontaneity. The
other side effect to watch out for is hypothyroidism, which may
develop insidiously. Body weight should be measured and thyroid and
renal function determined before starting lithium therapy and
annually thereafter.

8.11

Is lithium safe in pregnancy?

Women who are contemplating pregnancy should not take lithium
because of the risk of birth defects, especially cleft palate.

8.12

What are the important drug interactions of lithium?

Thiazide diuretics reduce the excretion of lithium and can result in
lithium toxicity. Neuroleptics, especially haloperidol, can cause rare

neurotoxicity with ataxia, confusion and hyper-reflexia as well as coma. This is more likely to occur when the drugs are given in high doses for acute mania while the patient is in hospital. Antidepressants, especially the SSRIs and anticonvulsants, can also potentiate the toxic effects of lithium.

8.13

Which patients are likely to benefit from long-term prophylaxis?

It is important to distinguish between the recurrence of depression when treatment is stopped too soon after an acute episode and recurrent illness in someone prone to frequent new episodes. Acute episodes should be treated for 4 to 6 months after full remission of all symptoms. Long-term prophylaxis should always be considered in those who have three distinct episodes in 2 years. Factors to consider are the severity of the illness and its social impact on the patient, the likelihood of the patient complying with long-term treatment and the quality of remission induced by therapy as well as the impact of side effects. Also to be taken into account are social and psychological factors, such as environmental stress, and life events, such as bereavements, which can act as triggers in vulnerable individuals. It should be borne in mind that the illness tends to get worse with recurrent episodes.

8.14

Is there a place for a mixture of pharmacological treatment and cognitive therapy in the long-term treatment of depression and the prevention of relapse?

There is evidence that interpersonal therapy, either alone or in combination with antidepressant medication, may delay relapses and improve social functioning in those who recover from depressive illnesses. Theoretically, cognitive therapy, either in the acute phase or when the patient is well, should enable patients to cope with and treat depressive episodes themselves, and even reduce their occurrence. Cognitive therapy is probably more appropriate at the milder end of the depressive spectrum where social, psychological and personality factors have a stronger part to play in the genesis of the depression/unhappiness. Maintenance medication is superior to psychological therapies for reducing relapse rates. The combination of cognitive therapy plus medication looks attractive but needs further evaluation.

PSYCHOTHERAPY AND COMPLEMENTARY MEDICINE

Introduction

Psychotherapy has a fundamental role to play in the treatment of depression, ranging from offering simple support and advice to dealing with issues of loss, bereavement, negative self-image and negative cognitions, poor self-esteem and all the other pathological patterns of thinking and behaviour that can result in depressive symptoms. At a deeper level, psychoanalytic psychotherapy deals with the exploration of early loss that results in patients experiencing current day situations as emotionally depressive. It is appropriate to combine psychotherapy with pharmacological treatments.

Anxiety states benefit from cognitive therapy to correct false interpretations of symptoms and to help patients cope with their symptoms. Anxiety management is a more elaborate process combining several therapeutic strategies.

Complementary medicines are increasingly employed as an alternative or adjunct to traditional therapies. Their nature makes formal evaluation difficult, although many people claim to benefit considerably from them.

PSYCHOTHERAPIES

9.1

Are regular counselling sessions for patients with long-standing depressive illness beneficial or do they encourage dependence?

Supportive psychotherapy, even when there is the feeling that nothing changes, is a greatly underrated treatment which offers a lifeline to many people. Dependency is not necessarily a bad thing, and patients usually lose their dependency on the GP when they get better. It may be that they need to depend on someone for a period of time, or even indefinitely, as a crutch to get them through. Seeing someone for brief periods of time every couple of weeks is a cost-effective treatment. If these sessions were stopped, many of these patients would find someone else who might handle the situation less well (or better). Others would undergo unnecessary investigations and the therapeutic alliance would need to be re-established. Depressed patients may deteriorate if they are no longer seen on a regular basis and it will take hard work to get them back to the baseline again. The danger is that, if a patient is seen too frequently, or for too long a period of time at each interview over too long a period of time, a transference relationship will take place in which he or she will develop unreasonable and inexplicable expectations of the therapist which relate to an infantile psychopathology, and which can be hard to deal with. The GP may be at risk of counter-transference, in some way reflecting unfulfilled emotional needs onto the patient, thus becoming dependent on the patient's continued reliance. It is important to be alert to these aspects of the psychotherapeutic relationship. They are not necessarily bad, but need to be recognized and dealt with, in which case they can be a great power for good and change.

9.2

How do I select the best of the possible treatments for an anxious patient?

The best approach offers patients help on a graduated basis, starting with simple interventions and building up to more complex ones. The initial intervention should involve a history and general counselling. It should work from establishing a clear definition of the problem and encouragement to adopt an active problem-solving method rather than a passive one. Counselling involves listening more than talking, but often nothing more complex than a sympathetic hearing and general practical advice.

If this fails, a more structured psychological intervention may be appropriate, which includes directive (straightforward advice) and non-directive counselling (encouraging the patient to work out the answer). Assertiveness training, relaxation and psychotherapy, anxiety management and cognitive therapy may be used. The choice of therapy depends upon availability of therapists and the appropriateness for the individual problem. Many of these therapies can be provided by a GP. Despite their grand names they are relatively simple. It should be possible to make a significant intervention over a series of three of four interviews, lasting 10 to 15 minutes.

If this approach fails, or is inappropriate, one may consider drug therapy. Benzodiazepines are only appropriate for the short-term treatment of anxiety, although for this they are quite effective. Antidepressants are also useful if patients are depressed, or present with chronic anxiety or panic. Buspirone is suitable for the management of generalized anxiety, and beta-blockers are sometimes useful when physical symptoms predominate.

When these measures fail, the GP may consider referral to a specialist. It is important to choose a specialist with appropriate experience and to make the reason for referral clear (Table 9.1).

Table 9.1 Four stages in the graduated approach of therapies	
1. Initial intervention	Simple counselling, listening, reassurance and advice
2. Psychological management	Formal psychological therapy support from community psychiatric nurse or practice counsellor
3. The use of medication	Short courses of: benzodiazepines; beta-blockers; antidepressants (buspirone)
4. Specialist care	Hospital specialist or trained clinical psychologist

9.3

How can the efficacy of psychological treatments be assessed?

The more analytical psychotherapies are hard to evaluate scientifically because they deal more with the process of change and general well-being and letting people sort out their own minds than with specific symptoms. There is impressive evidence to show that cognitive therapies and behavioural treatments are effective for the treatment of phobias, anxiety and depression, using measures such as symptom reduction, less use of therapists' time, etc. There is also the evidence of the GP's own experience of seeing patients get better and claiming benefit from the treatment. There is much evidence that shows that psychological treatments are as effective as pharmacological treatments for mild symptoms, although for more severe symptoms pharmacological treatments are probably better. The combination of the two treatments is probably best overall (Table 9.2).

Table 9.2 Psychological treatments for different anxiety disorders

Anxiety disorder	Psychological treatment
Acute stress reaction	Counselling
Specific phobias	Systematic desensitization
Generalized anxiety	Anxiety management training
Panic attacks	Cognitive therapy

9.4

Do day hospitals perpetuate the mental ill health/depression role?

Day hospitals and day centres fulfil several roles beyond being just somewhere to go and sit and share one's problems. They offer assessment whereby the functional skills and deficits of patients with mental illnesses can be assessed and addressed and therapeutic programmes designed to deal with these problems. They allow the patients to be observed in a structured environment so that a clearer understanding of the patient's problem can be gained. One of the worst problems of depression is that patients have a relatively unstructured lifestyle, and regular attendances at therapeutic programmes at least give some structure to a day which would otherwise be filled with emptiness and self-pity. The therapeutic programmes would then offer reality-based therapy, where patients would be encouraged to challenge their own depressive cognitions and have them replaced with more positive thoughts. They would be offered other forms of group therapy, and relaxation treatment aimed not only at dealing with false perceptions related to depression but also at thinking through the problems in their homes and outside lives which may have precipitated and maintained their depressions. Listening to other patients is often useful in making them realize that they are not alone in their situation. Often, seeing mistakes other people have made in their lives helps them realize they are making the same ones themselves. Other patients are often better at challenging an individual's false cognitions than staff, who are seen as being on the other side of the fence. Patients tend to complain about the worthless nature of day-care programmes, partly because of their general inability to engage with therapy and because of their depressive cognitions. As they become involved in programmes, and the programmes are more individually designed for them, they generally derive greater benefit from them.

9.5

Which sorts of patients should be referred for psychoanalysis?

Psychoanalysis is a complex therapy which explores patients' feelings about the world around them through their relationship with their therapist over a period of some time. It requires regular sessions, possibly once or twice or up to 5 times a week over a period of years. As such, it requires a degree of integration on behalf of the patient to sustain a long-term relationship, and to turn up and pay for regular sessions. Patients must be able to understand the meaning of the therapy and to tolerate some degree of stress when confronting their own painful memories and misconceptions about themselves and the world around them. Thus, not all patients are suitable to embark upon analytic therapy.

159

Classically, patients who do well are young, verbal, intelligent and single. They are people who still have the capacity to learn and change over a period of time, and who have the personal resources to work at their problem. Psychoanalysis works best for people with recurrent problems in their relationships with others. These individuals can explore their feelings via the problems they develop in their relationship with their therapist. In learning about themselves and how they view the world, they can gradually change their attitudes. It is not a panacea to get to the root problem of all ills, and understanding the cause does not necessarily lead to the cure.

9.6

What is the difference between psychoanalysis and psychotherapy?

Apart from the obvious differences of depth, cost and length of treatment, psychoanalysis is to do with understanding the self and resolving unconscious conflicts, thereby affecting change. Psychotherapy is much more to do with problem-solving as a treatment. People undergoing analysis are not necessarily ill, whereas therapy implies some measure of pathology which requires treatment. Psychotherapy can be almost any form of talking treatment, ranging from one or two simple sessions of counselling up to twice-weekly therapy for a year or two. Analysis is a highly specific and structured process.

9.7

What are the criteria for providing psychotherapy?

Psychotherapy is a wide concept which basically involves talking treatments, possibly through the mechanism of a therapeutic relationship. At its simplest level, it uses the relationship of trust between the doctor and the patient for the doctor to provide reassurance, empathy and explanation, and allows the patient to verbalize fears and concerns. It should, at this level, form the basis of every therapeutic encounter, whether or not other treatments are also used.

When dealing with more specific therapies, it is useful to consider what the goals of the therapy are, and to try to match the nature of the problem to the approach used. For example, an acute situational crisis may benefit from simple counselling; specific phobias call for systematic desensitization and graded exposure; generalized anxiety responds to relaxation training, reassurance and explanation; panic attacks are treated by cognitive therapy. Obsessive compulsive disorder is best treated with thought-stopping and response prevention. Not all problems are amenable to psychotherapy, despite patients' wishes. Severe depression should be treated with antidepressants as a first-line treatment since the patient will not be accessible to psychological interventions. Group therapy is often better than individual therapy, especially in those who use mechanisms of denial since the group can bring a unique collective pressure to bear. Many patients, for narcissistic reasons, want individual therapy, which is reserved for the most disturbed patients.

9.8

How can patients find a good therapist?

There are many different approaches to psychotherapy. Lists of suitably qualified therapists can be found through the National Register of Hypnotherapists and Psychotherapists, the British Association of Counsellors and the British Association of Psychotherapists, as well as through the Group Analytic Association and Relate. From a patient's point of view, the names of several therapists should be offered. Patient and therapist will be establishing a long-term relationship which is crucial for the therapy, and it is important that they can get on personally. The local consultant psychiatrist can offer an opinion and will know of several therapists and their particular suitability for the individual patient. He or she may also be able to 'prescribe' psychotherapy, in which case some health insurance companies would be prepared to pay the costs if the patient has health insurance.

9.9

What is the significance of different psychotherapeutic approaches?

Therapists may label themselves Freudian, Jungian, Kleinian, etc. The main difference is the symbolic language that the therapist uses, but all the analytic therapists would be working at the unconscious level. There would be differences in the structure of the therapy, but since these therapies at an analytical level rely on the relationship between patient and therapist to create an understanding of the underlying conflicts, and thereby to effect change, it is almost the relationship between the therapist and patient which is more important than the type of therapy.

9.10
What do patients need to know about their prospective therapist?

As well as the qualifications of the therapist and the experience within the relevant area, it would be useful to know the orientation of the therapist – whether they are analytically orientated and looking at the underlying problem, or, for example, cognitive behavioural therapists dealing more with a specific problem and the way the patient perceives and handles it. It is important to know the duration of the treatment and the frequency of sessions, and if the patient is being seen privately, then of course the cost is important. The most important factor, however, is that the patient feels able to establish a rapport with the therapist.

9.11
What protection do patients have when referred to psychotherapists who practise privately?

It is important for the GP to know the therapist personally, or at least by reputation, and to follow the patient up on a regular basis to ensure that things are progressing appropriately. It is useful to have several therapists available. Patients may be advised to have initial consultations with at least two therapists so that they can see if they will get on with them. Patients should be advised to come back to their GP if they are not happy about any aspect of their therapy. If there are problems, the GP should discuss them with the therapist before advising any patient to terminate; it is not unusual, as psychotherapy progresses, for patients to develop transference problems with their therapist which will make them want to drop out of therapy, as a feature of resistance, rather than to work through these problems, which is crucial to the success of therapy.

9.12

Can drugs and psychotherapy be used together effectively?

The best results are probably obtained by a combination of treatments. Some psychoanalysts feel that patients need symptoms in order to drive the therapeutic process. In these cases, relieving symptoms by medication may well be counterproductive. It may also be true of anxiety management, where patients should be desensitizing themselves to their symptoms and learning to cope with them rather than avoiding them. If they have no symptoms then they cannot learn how to deal with them. In patients with severe depression, psychotherapy probably has little part to play, and may in some cases be counterproductive by allowing them to torture themselves with their depressive preoccupations, or feeding into their depressive thoughts. Medication may make the patient more accessible to the therapist. In milder states, medication alone may prove ineffective.

9.13

How does brief focal therapy differ from other, more traditional forms?

This therapy is thought to be the most appropriate form of psychotherapy for use in general practice. It is more symptom-orientated than problem-orientated, and with a limited number of sessions. Ultimately it may be as effective for a given problem as longer therapies and it is certainly cheaper. The disadvantage is that it may not deal with the underlying problem causing the distress.

9.14

What are the features that makes this form of counselling suitable for use in general practice?

It is a relatively simple form of treatment which does not work on a deep psychoanalytical level, and should be suitable for a sympathetic

GP to apply. It offers a simple framework in which patients are asked to explore their problems and they themselves do the work in finding solutions. The therapist's role is to ask an appropriate question when an issue has been defined.

9.15

What is Rogerian counselling?

This is a non-directive form of therapy described by Carl Rogers, who stated that the most important qualities of a therapist were empathy, warmth and understanding. The therapy is client-centred and the client is in control of what is discussed; the counsellor helps the client work out ways of dealing with problems in a better way by listening, answering questions and trying to understand, and then reflecting back, for example by rephrasing what the client has said in a more sympathetic and understanding way. If a client says that there is a problem in dealing with his or her boss, the therapist would respond with the question, 'Why do you think you have troubles dealing with your boss?', which would require the client to explore the issue further. No direct advice or interpretation is given, and the aim of the counselling is to get clients to change their perceptions and attitudes. At the end of therapy, in the example used here, the client would understand better the relationship with his or her boss and the emotional impact of the difficulty would be understood and reduced.

9.16

How do the dynamics of group therapy differ from those of individual psychotherapy?

Apart from the obvious factor that seeing patients in groups is more cost-effective in terms of the therapist's time, groups have real advantages over individual therapy. For example, social skills groups enable patients to learn from others and role-play their social phobias in the presence of others. Groups are good for dealing with family dynamics, and isolated people often do well in groups. Anxiety management groups enable people to model their behaviour on others and dependency is dealt with better in a group situation than individually. Individual treatment is reserved for more intensive analytical-type psychotherapy and often as a prelude to getting people ready for longer-term group therapy. It is particularly useful for isolated autistic and borderline-type personalities.

9.17

Who should be referred to a behavioural therapist?

Behaviour therapy is particularly useful for problems which manifest themselves in undesirable behaviour – for example, for phobias where patients become anxious in specific situations – and where patients are otherwise relatively normal. It is also useful for problems such as toilet training in children, social interaction (e.g. social skills) and for eliminating socially undesirable behaviour (such as nail-biting) using reward. Aversion techniques are not used these days. Behaviour therapy works best when the problem is easily identifiable and relatively discrete, is quantifiable and quite frequent, such as school refusal. It works less well on diffuse problems which occur infrequently and unpredictably. The behavioural approach in many ways applies common sense (if you fall off a horse, get on again quickly before you lose your nerve) and can be learned from books or even computer programmes. It probably works best together with a cognitive component, allowing patients to think as well as do, in overcoming their problem, in the above example, offering an explanation about the finer techniques of horsemanship and saying that everybody falls off a horse from time to time, before getting back on again after a fall.

9.18

What is cognitive behaviour therapy?

Cognitive behaviour therapy is based on the principle that a person's mood and behaviour reflect the way he or she thinks, or, conversely, that moods are created by 'cognitions' or thoughts. It is therefore a therapeutic technique in which patients are encouraged to recognize negative patterns of thinking and to identify the links between negative thoughts, mood and behaviour. This encourages them to challenge these thoughts and replace them with more appropriate and reasonable perceptions.

165

9.19

What type of problem responds to cognitive therapy?

This is an effective therapy for problems in which there is an identifiable abnormality of thought process that results in anxiety or depression. The patient misperceives stimuli or events and interprets them as anxiety-provoking or distressing. The patient may process information selectively or overgeneralize. For example, a patient may assume, quite wrongly, that he or she is much less clever than everyone else at work. This results in feelings of inadequacy and depression. Treatment helps the patient examine the false premise about his or her stupidity by comparing various achievements with those of his or her colleagues and by looking at his or her work performance compared with others' in a rational way. It would also deal with any objections to this approach which might arise, by asking the patient to form a rational analysis of the facts. Another example would be a patient who misinterpreted a rapid heart beat as symptomatic of serious heart disease and impending death, rather than a normal physiological response to stress. The treatment would involve explanation of the physiology of heart rate, reasoned discussion about life expectancy and the improbability of sudden death in someone without manifest disease, and an exploration of other reasons for taking the worst possible scenario approach to a relatively trivial event.

9.20

What makes family therapy a useful approach in general practice?

This therapeutic approach enables the whole family to be treated as a functional, or dysfunctional unit, instead of as separate individuals. It is used to treat specific issues in a dynamic way, rather like brief focal psychotherapy. It has the advantage that the GP knows the whole family and sees the problem as arising from family dynamics, as opposed to isolating an individual who is identified as the sick member. For example, if a woman is depressed because her husband is having affairs and her children are deviant, then this would be seen as a family problem rather than simply regarding the woman as sick and treating her with antidepressants.

Sessions are held at longer intervals, perhaps every 4 to 6 weeks instead of weekly.

9.21

When is art therapy useful?

This form of therapy is particularly useful for patients who are unable to verbalize their problems, either because they are severely blocked and incapable or, for example in the case of children, because they do not possess the vocabulary to express themselves properly. It allows unconscious messages to come through to the conscious.

9.22

When is psychodrama a useful tool?

The technique of using role-playing to re-enact emotionally charged events offers a quick way to get in touch with grief and traumatic experiences. It needs a skilled therapist.

ANXIETY MANAGEMENT

9.23

What is anxiety management and what does it involve?

Anxiety management is a treatment consisting of several components which are designed to be used together to help patients deal with symptoms of anxiety. There is an educational component, explaining the nature and consequences of anxiety and the physiological mechanisms involved in the causation of bodily symptoms and fears. Patients are asked to undertake self-monitoring of symptoms, keeping diary cards to help them establish links between the internal and external environment. It has a cognitive component which encourages patients to think about and evaluate the fears and abnormal thoughts which give rise to their symptoms. It may have a behavioural

167

component, in which patients undergo systematic exposure to a phobic situation or object. Practical advice on new ways of coping and general support are also given. Progressive muscular relaxation is also an essential component, and other more specific techniques, such as bringing photos of particular significance to the sessions and talking about them, may be appropriate. The exact mix of techniques depends on the needs of the patient and the training of the therapist.

9.24

How is the diary card used in anxiety management?

The patient should be encouraged to draw up a daily prospective anxiety diary card (Fig. 9.1) which is used to chart the nature and severity of symptoms, their time and circumstances. Thoughts and attitudes connected with an increase or decrease in symptoms and coping strategies should be included.

Patients should be encouraged to explore the triggers both physical and psychological in as much detail as possible.

It is important to look for avoidance, either obvious or subtle, and also to detail both the physical and psychological components of the anxiety experienced. Associated with this, the patient should be helped to explore the consequences, for example, developing escape reactions or seeking reassurance. After this, it might be appropriate to investigate the underlying attitudes and beliefs concerning the anxiety

Time	Severity of symptom score 0 – 5	Main symptoms	Precipitant	Action
7 – 10				
10 – 2				
2 – 6				
6 – 12				

Figure 9.1 Example of a patient diary card to be filled in daily. It will demonstrate that symptoms can change in severity as a result of external events.

and its implications. A full life history is always essential, wider issues in the patient's life could be examined, including job satisfaction, marital and interpersonal relationships, sexual satisfaction and existential issues including 'the meaning of life' to the patient. Life structure is important for comparing the balance between work and personal life, exercise, diet and the use of substances such as alcohol, tobacco, tea, coffee and cola drinks.

Diary cards have the great virtue of making the patient do all the work. Writing all this down helps them work out the problem themselves.

9.25

How can the technique of deep muscular relaxation be used in the management of anxiety disorders?

This simple technique, which can be taught by almost anybody, or even by means of an anxiety management tape, involves learning how to relax the body and muscles. The patient simply lies or sits in a relaxed fashion and concentrates on tensing and then relaxing various muscle groups starting with the feet and gradually moving up the body, thereby learning the difference between tension and relaxation. The technique must be practised regularly, and patients must learn to use it at times when they are feeling tense. It can be used as a focus for an anxiety management group, run by a practice counsellor. It is of particular benefit to patients who have somatic symptoms, and who often fail to make the link between emotions and bodily feelings.

9.26

How effective are relaxation techniques in treating anxiety?

Simply handing a patient an anxiety management cassette, which is tried once or twice, is probably no more effective than giving a placebo which, of course, we know is highly effective. For relaxational techniques to be effective they have to be used frequently, probably once or twice a day over a period of time. Patients have to train for relaxation, in the same way that they train for physical fitness, rather than trying to relax once or twice and then giving up.

Deep muscle relaxation is best used in conjunction with an anxiety management package, forming an integral part of the treatment programme. Such programmes are quite effective at the milder end of the spectrum, especially in the hands of a skilled therapist. Some patients are so anxious, however, that they are unable to relax. At this point they may well benefit from some form of anxiolytic agent for a limited period before they are able to learn to relax, which is a technique they should use for the next stage of treatment.

9.27

Which relaxation tapes should patients use?

There are many different tapes available from health food shops, magazines and specialist mail order. Those that simply offer relaxation are probably less effective than those dealing with a more cognitive approach, giving specific advice on dealing with particular problems. The most effective relaxation tapes are those made individually for patients by their therapists after a session which are then used as homework.

9.28

What is hypnosis?

Hypnosis is a technique which places the patient in a profound state of relaxation in order for him or her to become suggestible at a subliminal level. It is not possible to make patients do things they do not want to do, but it helps them achieve certain psychological goals if they wish them to happen. It uses techniques of dissociation and was therefore originally used in the treatment of hysteria. During hypnosis patients can have certain suggestions placed in their minds, such as coughing whenever they light a cigarette. Or they may be enabled to relive traumatic past events, or to visualize phobic situations, while relaxed. They may imagine themselves in tranquil and beautiful settings to enhance the relaxation process. During this state the mind remains alert while the body is deeply relaxed. This allows emotionally charged memories to be uncovered and explored.

9.29

How can hypnotherapy bring things out of the unconscious into the conscious so that they can be dealt with?

If a problem is defined in a hypnotic trance at a subconscious level, and the situation can be dealt with at that level, then theoretically this should result in the resolution of the conflict, thereby affecting a cure in the conscious. This line of reasoning requires a highly mechanistic view of the functioning of the mind and presupposes a separation of conscious and unconscious levels. A more reasonable view would be that problems can be explored while the individual is relaxed, and the emotional impact of unresolved conflict is thereby gradually desensitized.

9.30

What sort of problems benefit from hypnosis?

Hypnosis works via suggestion at a subliminal level. Originally, in the 19th century hypnosis was used as a treatment for hysteria, but this is a very rare and dangerous condition to diagnose. Because it works via suggestion at a subliminal level, it is useful for anxiety states when patients can relax themselves using a technique very similar to standard relaxation techniques and progressive muscular relaxation. It helps patients relive and re-enact repressed trauma in a controlled way, thus enabling a resolution of conflicts and anxieties. It can be used as a form of desensitization in the imagination for phobic patients who can approach their feared objects while in a relaxed, disassociated state. In all these conditions, hypnosis works in a similar fashion to non-hypnotic techniques for dealing with the problem, but because of the additive effect of suggestion and relaxation, progress can be faster and more profound than without hypnosis.

Hypnosis is of particular value in pain management, either in acute situations such as in dental treatment, or for chronic pain where patients can alter their focus of attention and disassociate from the pain, possibly by some functional change in the nervous system. In the treatment of smoking addiction and eating disorders, hypnosis can have an additive effect on the patient's own resolve by the power of suggestion. However, there are also problems with hypnosis. Despite dramatic demonstrations of its power and popularity among its protagonists, demonstrating clinical efficacy remains a problem. Some patients develop a strong attachment to their therapist and only a limited proportion of patients are good subjects for hypnosis.

COMPLEMENTARY MEDICINE

9.31

Is acupuncture effective in the treatment of anxiety or depression?

Acupuncture is not particularly helpful for anxiety and depression.

9.32

Have any of the other alternative therapies, such as reflexology, aromatherapy or shiatsu, been shown to work in depression and/or anxiety?

The proponents of these therapies and those who make use of them claim considerable benefit in emotional well-being and the resolution of anxiety and depression. These therapies are particularly appropriate for patients whose lifestyles would benefit from a more holistic approach to their symptoms and problems. There is, of course, no hard data to support this view, but I am sure these therapies work for some people.

9.33

What about herbal remedies for depression, in particular St John's Wort – hypericum? It is claimed that it relieves depression and is, I believe, widely used in Europe. I understand that there have been few controlled trials.

A recently published meta-analysis in the *British Medical Journal* showed that hypericum was more effective than placebo in treating depression. Claims that it was as effective as antidepressants were unfounded since there have been no controlled trials comparing hypericum to a proper dose of antidepressants. It seems to help in mild depression and some patients prefer a natural remedy.

9.34

Are there any homeopathic remedies for depression and/or anxiety?

There are certainly homeopathic remedies available, but homeopathy is a complex area which does not lend itself to simple prescription of a compound in order to effect a cure. Whether any of these remedies is more effective than placebo remains in doubt. The efficacy of the remedy will be in proportion to the commitment that the person makes to the process – beyond that I am not qualified to comment.

9.35

What steps can a depressed patient take to help him- or herself?

Patients should be encouraged to talk about their fears and feelings, and to keep as active as possible. It is important that they eat despite having no appetite, and they should avoid alcohol since it is a bad self-medicant. If they experience sleep disturbance they should not fret about it, and should reassure themselves that they will get better. They should see their doctor or therapist and comply with treatment recommendations.

9.36

Is there anything that friends or relatives can do to help?

They should offer a sympathetic ear without criticism, showing warmth and empathy. They should encourage the patient in his or her own endeavours and offer companionship and reassurance. Relatives should try to ensure that patients do not drink to excess or take illicit drugs.

10 SUICIDE AND PARASUICIDE

Introduction

The reduction of suicide rates has been one of the key targets in the British government's 'Health of the Nation' statement (1992 Health of the Nation, HMSO, London). Suicidal patients are usually seen by a doctor in the weeks before death but generally go unrecognized. The epidemic of suicide attempts continues unabated and is almost taken for granted – people at risk can be identified, but the actual prevention of suicide remains more of a problem.

10.1

How can GPs assess suicidal intent – or risks – in the depressed patient?

Most depressed patients will admit to some suicidal ideation but it is the level of ideation which is important. For example, if the patient has made plans and already acted on them, such as working out what the lethal dose of medication is and taking steps to obtain it, and is now just waiting for one event, such as his wife going away, to complete the act, this is a very high suicide risk. Simply wondering whether life is really worth living at a philosophical level can be regarded as low risk. Patients generally welcome being asked about suicidal intention and doctors should not be frightened of asking about it. It does not put the idea into the patient's head. Patients often feel relieved to discuss their worst fears. From a statistical point of view, people at particular risk are elderly, depressed males who have alcohol problems and are socially isolated. They feel hopeless and often have physical illness. Having a medical background is also a risk factor. In simple terms, an elderly, widowed, depressed doctor with a terminal illness and socially isolated, has the means of killing him- or herself and is at considerable risk. Another group at high risk for suicide includes young psychotic patients who appear to be recovering and in whom insight is returning. For both groups the greatest risk of suicide is at a time when they make a partial recovery. Their energy level increases but their sense of despair remains, and this combination of events makes them particularly vulnerable.

Most people who kill themselves have contact with a doctor in the preceding weeks. People who ultimately kill themselves are often undertreated for their depression, having been given inadequate courses of antidepressants or none at all.

10.2

How common is suicide in the elderly?

Suicide statistics in general are difficult to interpret because of the problems in the way they are reported. They thus represent a gross underestimate of the true picture. The official figures for England and Wales are 121 suicides per million males, and 57 per million females. Suicide rates increase significantly in the elderly where attempts at self-harm are much more likely to be aimed at suicide than as a suicidal gesture. 8% of men and 3% of women who have made a suicide attempt when aged over 55 have been shown ultimately to kill themselves.

10.3

What can be done to prevent suicide in the elderly?

The vast majority of elderly suicide attempters are clinically depressed, so the most important preventive measure is to diagnose and treat their depression effectively. Most people who kill themselves are seen by a doctor in the weeks prior to their death. Thus, prompt medical, social and psychological treatment for their depressive states is important. Doctors should especially be aware of patients with significant self-neglect and those who abuse alcohol.

10.4

How can the patient who is depressed yet stable be distinguished from one who is depressed and may kill him- or herself?

The patient should be asked directly if he or she has any suicidal ideation or plans. The patient will usually be honest and relieved to have been asked the question. Some patients may be evasive and this should be taken as a danger sign. Clearly, the degree of nihilism and lack of hope for the future are important. Patients with impulsive personality disorders are quite likely to make attempts and sadly a small proportion may be successful. Those who have made previous attempts are at much higher risk at further attempts. Patients should be asked if they feel they have anything to live for.

10.5

If it appears that a patient is really suicidal, what should be done?

The patient should be admitted to hospital immediately. Unfortunately, except in extreme cases, suicidal patients rarely give real indications that they are about to harm themselves. People who take overdoses or make parasuicide attempts usually do it for some ulterior motive rather than actually to kill themselves. If there is a risk of suicide or suicide attempt, then prescriptions should be limited to one week's supply at a time of a safe antidepressant and the patient monitored carefully until there has been an adequate improvement in his or her clinical state. The people who kill themselves tend to be either elderly isolated males, or young psychotic patients who have the insight to realize that their future lives are grim and decide they no longer wish to carry on living. Family support is helpful in monitoring the situation. Unfortunately, it is often the silent, non-complaining person who commits suicide rather than the dramatic hysteric who projects all his anxieties onto the doctor and feels better him- or herself.

10.6

Is an overdose of antidepressants the commonest method of affecting suicide?

15% of patients with severe depressions ultimately kill themselves. Antidepressants, although frequently taken as overdoses, are rarely implicated – only about one patient a day in the UK dies in this way. This is about the same as those who die by using paracetamol. These figures have to be put in the context of about 4500 suicides per annum, thus antidepressant overdoses account for about 5% of all suicides. Lethal overdoses tend to be more common in urban communities, whereas violent methods such as hanging and shooting are more common in rural communities. Reducing suicide rates is one of the key tenets in the Health of the Nation document.

10.7

Should the number of pills prescribed to depressed patients be restricted in order to try to limit their use for suicide?

An important way to prevent suicide is to treat depression vigorously: many more patients die because of inadequately treated depression than because of taking antidepressant overdoses. The older tricyclic-type antidepressants are far more lethal in overdose than newer antidepressants such as the SSRIs and lofepramine. Very few, if any, deaths have occurred as a result of overdoses from these drugs alone. Thus, if there is suspicion of a suicidal risk in a depressed patient, the GP should encourage him or her to take a full dose of antidepressants, but the patient should probably be restricted to a couple of weeks' supply until the suicide risk has passed (at the same time ensuring he or she takes the medication in full doses).

10.8

What is parasuicide?

Parasuicide is suicidal-like behaviour, otherwise known as 'deliberate self-harm'. When dealing with these patients it soon becomes clear that, although they take an overdose or otherwise risk their lives, the real intention is not to kill themselves. Theirs is more of an impulsive act, a cry for help, an attempt at manipulating a situation. The intention to kill themselves is not very strong and therefore failed suicides are called parasuicides.

Parasuicide is about 15 times more common in men and 30 times more common in women than successful suicide. About 1 or 2% of parasuicides kill themselves within a 2-year period – a death rate some 50 to 100 times higher than that of the general population. The eventual death rate of people who indulge in parasuicide may be as high as 20% so it is not without risk.

10.9

What do you know about how the Samaritans selects and trains its telephone counsellors?

In the true self-help tradition, Samaritans used to be recruited from former suicide attempters. In recent years they have been taking a wider spread of counsellors who have not necessarily made suicide attempts themselves. They are trained by sitting in on counselling sessions and are later supervised by more experienced Samaritans. The Samaritans' national telephone helpline number is 0345 909090. Telephone numbers for local branches appear in the telephone directory. The organization offers round-the-clock help to thousands of desperate people.

GENERAL MANAGEMENT ISSUES

Introduction

The more treatable anxiety and depression become, the more doctors are advised to look for treatable aspects in an individual patient's problem. Repeated exposure to attractive therapeutic options by advertising can increase the inclination to diagnose conditions to apply them to. Doctors want to be as helpful as possible. Armed with the medical model of health, social ills tend to be medicalized. Doctors sometimes develop feelings of omnipotence; perhaps they can deal with almost all the problems that are presented to them. The counter argument is, of course, that depression is underdiagnosed and undertreated. There is probably no harm in a therapeutic trial if appropriate, providing it is also acknowledged that a trial of antidepressants, for example, should be stopped after a month if there is no demonstrable benefit.

The difference between depression and unhappiness ultimately comes down to a question of severity and treatability, together with the degree of social disability, that should influence therapeutic intervention.

11.1

How do anxiety and depression affect general health?

If anxiety and depression are primary conditions, then secondary disturbances, such as eating disorders, increased alcohol consumption and excessive smoking, arise as a consequence of the underlying disorder. On the other hand, people with primary eating disorders, alcohol dependency and a limited lifestyle often get mild depression and anxiety. Clearly, a healthy lifestyle is important for emotional well-being, but the relationship between the primary and secondary conditions needs to be explored. Exercise is one important element, since regular exercise improves health, well-being and mood, and few patients get enough exercise.

11.2

Is there any evidence that placebos work in the treatment of depression and anxiety?

Up to 50% of any response to the best therapeutic agents in this area is a placebo response, and in general practice this placebo response rate may be even higher. For example, antidepressants give approximately a 70% improvement rate, and the placebo response rate is between 30 and 50%. Added to this is the spontaneous remission rate. This is an area which is poorly understood, but it is an observable phenomenon that the level of conviction a doctor has in the benefits of treatment will affect the clinical outcome in the patient. Placebo responses are seen in many therapeutic areas.

11.3

Why, if anxiety is such a common complaint, do GPs have difficulty handling it?

Some estimates put the incidence of anxiety in general practice attendances as high as 15%. GPs recognize about 60% of anxiety disorders. The main reason for missing the remainder is that many patients present with the somatic features of anxiety, or with conditions where physical symptoms are predominant and the anxiety component may well appear to be secondary to the physical illness. Thus the doctor will tend to focus on the physical complaint. Other patients are reluctant to talk in terms of emotional complaints and use somatic complaints as an entry point to the consultation in the hope, conscious or unconscious, that the GP will probe and find clues as to the underlying causes. Another reason is that doctors are keen not to miss a physical condition, whereas, missing an emotional problem is regarded as far less serious. Finally, many anxiety-related disorders are genuine conditions, but often of a relatively minor nature and self-limiting and have a generally good prognosis whether or not they are recognized by the doctor. As a rule, however, anxiety disorders benefit from being recognized and treated.

11.4

What proportion of GP consultations are for depression?

Depression is a common complaint. 5% of patients consulting their GP show signs of major depression. Another 5% have minor depression and a further 10% show some depressive symptoms. At least one patient with depression is likely to present at each surgery. In a year a GP will treat about 3% of the people on his or her list for depression and about the same proportion will present with masked forms which may not be diagnosed. Perhaps up to 50% of patients seen by GPs have underlying psychological problems, although not all of these have definable depressive or other psychological illnesses (Table 11.1).

Table 11.1 Approximate prevalence rates (%) of depression

–	Point prevalence	One year	Life
Major	3	4	10
Dysthymia	2	3	15
Bipolar	1	1	1
Recurrent brief		6	

11.5

Is the willingness of depressed patients to be admitted to hospital an indication of the magnitude of their depression?

The main indicator of the severity of depression is the functional impairment. If a patient is so ill that he or she can no longer be maintained at home and requires inpatient care, this would indicate severe depression.

Other factors which influence hospital admission are the level of social support available outside hospital and the availability of hospital inpatient beds. For example, patients in private practice tend to find it easier to get admitted to hospital than do those fighting their way into an inner city NHS hospital bed.

Reasons for admitting patients should include concern about suicidal risk, patients not feeding themselves properly, and the need for inpatient ECT. A common reason for admitting a patient is a lack of insight and poor compliance with medication, either because of side effects or through inability to co-operate with treatment. In this case, a few days' inpatient care will establish a patient on a proper therapeutic regimen. Another reason for admitting patients with depression is if there are other comorbid psychiatric or physical problems.

11.6

Should we be referring more depressed patients to a specialist for advice and management?

The majority of depressed patients are seen by the GP, with the psychiatrist only seeing the tip of the iceberg. Referring more patients to your psychiatrist is impracticable, since it would swamp the services, and unnecessary, since GPs for the most part treat their patients appropriately. Most patients do not need referral and for the most part do not wish to be referred to a psychiatrist since it confirms their view that they are going mad.

Patients to be referred should include those about whose diagnosis there is some doubt, or who present with multiple pathology, those with severe depression or a risk of suicide, and those who might need ECT or specialist psychotherapy. Another group comprises patients

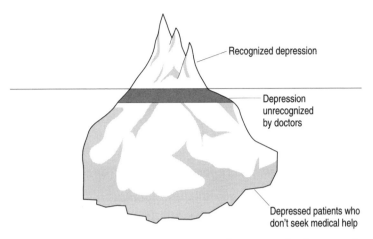

Fig. 11.1 The iceberg of depression. (From Kelly D 1987. The diagnosis of masked depression. In: Kelly D, France R (eds) A practical handbook for the treatment of depression. Parthenon Publishing, Lancashire.)

who have failed first-line treatments and those with whom the GP has a difficult relationship.

Ideally, the psychiatrist should visit the GP's practice from time to time, in order to discuss the management of depressed patients as part of a clinical case conference. This enables them to perceive difficulties and offer solutions to each other, since psychiatrists and GPs generally see a different population of patients (Fig. 11.1).

11.7

What proportion of a general psychiatrist's workload is concerned with depression?

A general psychiatrist in an inner city would find that about a half of all new outpatient appointments are to do with anxiety and depression. Half of these have depressive illnesses.

11.8

Why is it so difficult to diagnose depression?

The answer must lie in areas of lack of training and lack of time, but most importantly, in not considering it as a first diagnosis. Depression is often masked, presenting with somatic symptoms, and the difficulty always is deciding at which point to consider a psychological cause for the symptoms. Doctors are taught to exclude organic pathology before considering a psychological cause, but missing organic pathology is rare (if memorable). Missing a treatable depression is all too common.

11.9

Why do GPs fail to recognize 50% of depressed patients?

There appear to be some factors which hinder recognition of depressed patients. The obvious one is when depression co-exists with physical illness. Depressive illnesses can develop insidiously and be mistaken for a symptom of the physical illness. There are also difficulties in patients who present with physical complaints and somatization disorders which are commonly suspected of being organic in origin. Another problem arises in patients who have been depressed for some time, in whom depression is seen more as a characterological trait or life pattern than a depressive illness, and in whom a low mood is taken for granted. Problems can arise in those who express less overt or atypical symptoms, such as in ethnic minorities, who often somatize symptoms. It is also easy to miss the diagnosis in elderly people, in whom unhappiness is often confused with senility or a generally pessimistic outlook on life as families move away and friends die.

Characteristics in the doctor can influence diagnostic acumen. Those who make good eye contact with the patient are less likely to miss depressive disorders, and those who ask direct questions about psychological or social problems are more likely to get relevant answers than those who choose to gloss over the issues. Doctors who empathize, tolerate silence and are receptive to non-verbal behaviour are more likely to recognize depressive illnesses.

Older GPs and those working on their own tend to refer more patients to psychiatrists. It is hard to say whether this means that they actually diagnose more or simply refer those they do diagnose.

11.10

What are the implications of a missed diagnosis of depression?

Depression is a condition of high morbidity which is eminently treatable. 15% of patients with depression ultimately die by suicide. There are 4500 suicides per year in the UK, 70% of which are thought to be associated with depression. No less important is the morbidity associated with depression, which results in poor work performance or time off work. In the current economic climate, if someone is off work for an extended period they are likely to lose their job and may never find work again. If depression is missed and the patient is diagnosed wrongly, there is the cost and inconvenience of unnecessary investigations. Depression in a family member produces strains on the relationships as well as secondary damage in the form of alcoholism and other problems. If depression is recognized and treated, much of the morbidity and diminution of quality of life can be prevented.

11.11

Should other members of the practice team be trained to recognize depression?

District nurses and health visitors who visit patients in their homes probably spend more time with patients than do doctors. The former establish relationships with patients over a period of time and are therefore ideally suited to recognize depression. They may not be sensitized to thinking about the co-existence of depressive illnesses, and should be encouraged to consider whether they are missing something. If they suspect depression, they should inform the GP accordingly. The practice receptionist can also be a mine of information. There is a lot to be said for simple screening questionnaires such as HADS (Ch. 1), which takes about 3 minutes for the patient to fill out and gives a pretty reliable indication of whether he or she is depressed or anxious or in a borderline state. It should be used if a mood disturbance is suspected. It is certainly cheaper than sending off for a blood count if a patient complains of tiredness and more likely to yield important information.

187

11.12

What do people in general feel about depression and its treatment?

A recent MORI poll for the Defeat Depression campaign showed that 22% of people have experienced depression themselves and 55% have reported experiencing depression either personally or through a close friend or relative. Everyone agreed that anybody could suffer from depression and 25% believed that women were at greater risk than men. 60% felt that children could suffer from depression. Life events such as death, unemployment and divorce were seen as major causes, and about one-third of people felt that depression had a biological basis. Half of the people interviewed knew that postnatal depression could occur and a similar number knew of depression associated with the menopause.

78% of people believed that antidepressants were addictive. Half thought they were effective, but a third thought they were ineffective. 85% believed counselling was effective.

Over half felt the GP was the best person to consult if depressed, but again half felt that their GP would simply think them neurotic, and a quarter felt their GP would be irritated or annoyed. Thus, there remain considerable misconceptions in people's minds about depression and its treatment.

11.13

How can GPs improve their management of depression?

The first priority is to adopt a positive approach and convince patients that they have an illness which will get better with help and treatment. It is important for patients to consult one doctor who can then follow the patient up personally for several months and monitor progress. There should be a standard approach to the discussion and to record keeping to improve uniformity and completeness of records. There should be definite review appointments, since one of the major problems in the management of depression is poor compliance and failure to follow up. It is known that many patients are loathe to take antidepressant medication.

Because of the general feelings of unworthiness associated with depression, patients feel they are wasting their doctor's time, and, if the treatment is not immediately effective, they feel the doctor will be unable to help them. Even if treatment is effective, patients should be followed up for several months after the acute phase of the illness to monitor possible relapses, and to make sure they make a full recovery.

Psychological treatments – for example, counselling and cognitive therapy – should be considered either as first-line treatment, or when the immediate symptoms have been relieved by medication and the depression can be seen as a pattern of maladaptive psychological behaviour. In this case, patients should be encouraged to learn ways of avoiding future situations in which they are prone to developing depression.

Antidepressants should be prescribed in full doses for a minimum of 4 to 6 weeks and then reviewed formally, rather than half-heartedly prescribing an inadequate dose of antidepressants which the patient takes intermittently. The illness needs to be treated for an adequate length of time and the response to treatment reviewed. If a first-line treatment does not work, alternatives should be considered, such as a different antidepressant, psychological treatments or referral to a specialist.

Compliance is improved if patients understand their condition, and it may be helpful to include the relatives in an explanation of the condition. Self-help material about the nature of the condition and its treatment is also useful. It is also important to have good communication between therapists, GPs, counsellors, social workers, patients and other people involved in care so that miscommunication can be avoided.

11.14

What training is available to help GPs improve their diagnostic and management skills and the treatment offered to patients?

GP vocational training has improved the psychiatric skills of newer GPs who will be more skilled at interviewing patients. Training sessions could be arranged using video feedback, again to enhance interviewing skills. Good links should be encouraged with the local psychiatrist so that he or she can better understand the needs of GP colleagues (and strengths and weaknesses in dealing with patients can be assessed). Ideally, the psychiatrist should be encouraged to visit the practice and see a few patients in conjunction with the GP, so improving the skills of the GP and establishing a better relationship with the psychiatrist.

Continuing postgraduate education should be encouraged and audit and assessment should form part of clinical practice, in the presence of the local psychiatrist if possible.

11.15

Why do some patients engender feelings of helplessness or anger while others arouse great sympathy?

This is a common phenomenon which has been called counter-transference. It is a term derived from psychoanalytic thinking, where patients and the way they treat their therapist provoke emotions in the therapist which were reserved for key figures in childhood. The general demeanour of a complaining patient may well bring to mind a childhood situation associated with unexpressed anger. In a similar way, during the consultation angry feelings emerge but cannot be expressed because of the professional relationship.

It is important to recognize these emotions, which are not always negative. They may provide clues to the patient's underlying despair, helplessness or need to evoke sympathy in others because the patient probably arouses similar feelings in other people. They project their feelings onto their therapist. For example, some patients in their daily encounters make people angry because of the inadequacy they project. This compounds their problems in life by making them unpopular. If the therapist can face this and interpret it, it is the first step towards the patients' recognition of it in themselves, and possibly doing something about it.

In real life terms, all doctors have patients they get on with and those that they do not. If it is really a problem, it may be worth considering referring the patient on to someone else with a different set of internal values.

11.16

How can patients' feelings of despair be turned to good account?

Some patients communicate gloom by just sitting in the surgery and recounting how dreadful they feel. They are projecting their inner despair, which an experienced clinician is able to pick up. Problems can be expressed non-verbally as well as verbally. Unfortunately, the patient communicates a similar despair to everyone else and gets little back. The way to deal with it would be for doctors to confront the situation and tell the patient how dreadful they feel when they hear how dreadful the patient feels, which would be a way of making contact psychologically.

An alternative psychological approach would be to challenge the patient's maladaptive thinking pattern and the silent assumptions which underlie his or her depression. For example, patients may feel dreadful because they feel that no-one likes them. One could examine whether some people, such as close family and children, like them, whether you as their doctor like them, and how important it is for them to be liked. One could then examine what it is in such patients' behaviour that makes other people not like them. This would be the foundation of a cognitive behavioural approach.

11.17

How effective is the new group Depressives Anonymous, which relies on the 12-step approach, in the light of the fact that depression is not an addictive illness?

Depressives Anonymous is one of many 12-step organizations, although less well developed than Alcoholics Anonymous and Narcotics Anonymous. Unfortunately, depressed patients are less able to organize and sustain the work and commitment required to keep the meetings running so the organization has its problems.

11.18

How can a GP hope to offer sufficient counselling services when so many patients need them?

Some GPs have a particular interest in psychological therapies and may well choose to make time available for them – for example, one session a week. Otherwise, they can employ a practice counsellor, or even run groups in their surgery. Community psychiatric nurses may well supervise groups or act as counsellors. The GP may forge links with psychotherapeutic training establishments which can provide trainees under supervision to work in the practice. Research has shown that four to six 10-minute counselling sessions can be as effective as prescribing antidepressant or anxiolytic medication, and, although it may take slightly more time initially, it may well save time in the long term. In the new environment of the health service, GPs should be able to purchase more specialist psychotherapy from the clinical psychology services if so desired.

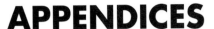

APPENDICES

Self help

Self-help material is particularly useful in anxiety and depression where patient information is so important. Leaflets are available from the Royal College of Psychiatrists, the BMA (*Coping with stress*), and many drug companies. Books can be obtained from bookshops and libraries. Patients should be recommended material appropriate to their level of functioning. Information is a key tenet of a cognitive behavioural approach, and patients need to know much more than can be conveyed in a short consultation. They also tend to forget so much of what they are told.

FURTHER READING

Anxiety and depression
Priest R 1996 Anxiety and depression. Century Vermilion, London
Shreeve C 1994 Overcoming depression: practical steps towards
    recovery. Thorsons, London
Weekes C 1995 Peace from nervous suffering. Thorsons, London
Weekes C 1995 Self help for your nerves. Thorsons, London

Phobias
Breton S 1996 Panic attacks: a practical guide to recognising and
    dealing with feelings of panic. Century Vermilion, London
Marks I 1995 Living with fear. McGraw-Hill, New York

Tranquillizers
Trickett S 1998 Coming off tranquillizers, sleeping pills and anti-
    depressants. Thorsons, London
Tranquillizer independence – self-help audio cassette from Dr Cosmo
    Hallstrom, the Charter Clinic, Chelsea, 7 Radnor Walk, London SW3
    4BP

Bereavement
Code of practice for Funeral Directors. From National Association of
    Funeral Directors, 618 Warwick Road, Solihull, West Midlands B91
    1AN

USEFUL ADDRESSES

Anxiety and depression

Age Concern Cymru
4th floor, 1 Cathedral Road
Cardiff CF1 9SD
Tel: 01222 371566 Fax: 01222 399562

Age Concern England
1268 London Road
London SW16 4ER
Tel: 0181 679 8000 Fax: 0181 679 6069

Age Concern Northern Ireland
3 Lower Crescent
Belfast BT7 1NR
Tel: 01232 245729 Fax: 01232 235497

Age Concern Scotland
113 Rose Street
Edinburgh EH2 3DT
Tel: 0131 220 3345 Fax: 0131 220 2779

Alzheimer's Disease Society
Gordon House
10 Greencoat Place
London SW1P 1PH
Tel: 0171 306 0606

Association for Post-Natal Illness
(APNI)
25 Jerdan Place
London SW6 1BE
Helpline: 0171 386 0868

CRY-SIS Support Group
BM CRY-SIS
London WC1N 3XX
Helpline: 0171 404 5011
(Support for parents with an
incessantly crying baby)

Depression Alliance
PO Box 1022
London SE1 7QB
Tel: 0171 633 9929

Depressives Anonymous
36 Chestnut Avenue

Beverley
North Humberside HU17 9QU
Tel: 01482 860619

Help the Aged
16–18 St James's Walk
London EC1R 0BE
Tel: 0171 253 0253 Fax: 0171 250 4474

Manic Depression Fellowship Ltd
8–10 High Street
Kingston upon Thames
Surrey KT1 1EY
Tel: 0181 974 6550 Fax: 0181 974 6600
Manchester office tel: 0161 953 4105
Caerleon office tel: 01633 430 353

Meet-a-Mum Association (MAMA)
26 Avenue Road
South Norwood
London SE25 4DX
Tel: 0181 771 5595
Helpline: 0181 768 0123
Monday–Friday 7.00pm–10.00pm

MIND
15–19 Broadway
London E15 4BQ
Admin tel: 0181 519 2122
Fax: 0181 522 1725
**National information line: 0345
660163**
Monday–Friday 9.15am–4.45pm
London callers: 0181 522 1728

National Association for
Premenstrual Syndrome (NAPS)
PO Box 72
Sevenoaks
Kent TN13 1QX
Tel: 01732 741709

National Childbirth Trust
Alexandra House
Oldham Terrace
London W3 6NH
Tel: 0181 992 8637 For local groups,
see local phone book

Royal College of Psychiatrists
17 Belgrave Square
London SW1X 8PG
Tel: 0171 235 2351

The Samaritans
10 The Grove
Slough
Berks SL1 1QP
Admin tel: 01753 532713 Fax: 01753 819004
National helpline: 0345 909090

Saneline
2nd floor, 199–205 Old Marylebone Road
London NW1 5QP
Admin tel: 0171 724 6520 or 724 8000
National helpline: 0345 678000
2.00pm–midnight daily
London callers: 0171 724 8000

Seasonal Affective Disorders Association (SADA)
PO Box 989
London SW7 2PZ
Tel: 01903 814942

Seasonal Affective Disorders Clinic
c/o Dr S. Checkley
The Maudsley Hospital
Denmark Hill
London SE5 8AZ
Tel: 0171 703 6333

Alcohol Abuse

Alcohol Concern
Waterbridge House
32–36 Lomas Street
London SE1 0EE
Tel: 0171 928 7377

Alcoholics Anonymous
PO Box 1
Stonebow House
Stonebow
York YO1 2NJ

Admin tel: 01904 644026 for information on UK offices
London helpline: 0171 352 3001
10.00am–10.00pm daily
For local branches, see local telephone book

Al-Anon Family Group
61 Great Dover Street
London SE1 4YF
Tel: 0171 403 0888

Alateen (a part of Al-Anon for young people whose families are affected by alcohol)
61 Great Dover Street
London SE1 4YF
Tel: 0171 403 0888

Drinkline
7th floor, Weddel House
13–14 West Smithfield
London EC1A 9DL
Helpline: 0345 320202
9.30am–11.00pm weekdays,
6.00pm–11.00pm weekends
24-hour dial-and-listen service: 0500 801 802
London callers: 0171 332 0202

National Association for Children of Alcoholics
PO Box 64
Fishponds
Bristol BS16 2YY
Helpline: 0800 289061
9.00am–5.00pm, Monday–Friday

Northern Ireland Community Addiction Service
40 Elmwood Avenue
Belfast BT9 6AZ
Tel: 01232 664434

Scottish Council on Alcohol
2nd floor, 166 Buchanan Street
Glasgow G1 2NH
Tel: 0141 333 9677

Young People

Advice, Advocacy and Representation
for Children
Canterbury House
1–3 Greengate
Salford M3 7NN
Helpline: 0800 616101
(For children in local authority / foster
care)

Anti-bullying Campaign
Admin tel: 0171 378 1446, office hours

Childline
Freepost 1111
London N1 0BR
National helpline: 0800 1111
24 hours
**Childline for Children in Care: 0800
88 4444**
daily 6.00pm–10.00pm

Childline Scotland
Freepost 1111
Glasgow G1 1BR
Helpline on bullying: 0800 44 1111
3.30pm–9.30pm, Monday–Friday

Children First
41 Polwarth Terrace
Edinburgh EH11 1NU
Admin tel: 0131 337 8539
Fax: 0131 346 8284

Kidscape
152 Buckingham Palace Road
London SW1W 9TR
Parents' advice line: 0171 730 3300
Bullying counsellor available
Tuesday, Wednesday, Thursday

National Children's Bureau
8 Wakely Street
London EC1V 7QE
Admin tel: 0171 843 6000

National Children's Home
85 Highbury Park
London N5 1UD
Admin tel: 0171 226 2033
Fax: 0171 226 2537

National Children's Home Scotland
17 Newton Place
Glasgow G3 7PY
Admin tel: 0141 332 4041
Fax: 0141 332 7002

National Children's Home Wales
St David's Court
68a Cowbridge Road East
Cardiff CF1 9DN
Admin tel: 01222 222127
Fax: 01222 229952

NSPCC Child Protection Helpline
(England, Wales and Northern
Ireland)
42 Curtain Road
London EC2A 3NH
Helpline: 0800 800 500

Northern Ireland Interlink Children's
Helpline
121 Spencer Road
Londonderry BT47 1AE
Helpline 0800 212 888 office hours

Parentline
Endway House
The Endway
Hadleigh
Essex SS7 2AN
UK helpline: 01702 559900
Monday–Friday 9.00am–9.00pm,
Saturday 1.00pm–6.00pm

Sexwise
Network Scotland
The Mews
57 Ruthven Lane
Glasgow G12 9JQ
National helpline: 0800 282930

Stepfamily – National Stepfamily
Association
72 Willesden Lane
London NW6 7TA
Admin tel: 0171 372 0844
Helpline: 0171 372 0846
Monday–Friday, 2.00pm–5.00pm,
7.00pm–10.00pm

Youthline (Northern Ireland)
2a Ribble Street
Belfast BT4 1HW
Helpline: 01232 456654
10.00am–10.00pm weekdays

Counselling/Psychotherapy

British Association for Counselling
(BAC)
1 Regent Place
Rugby
Warwickshire CV21 2PJ
Tel: 01788 578328

Westminster Pastoral Foundation
23 Kensington Square
London W8 5HN
Admin tel: 0171 937 6956
Fax: 0171 937 1767

Phobias

First Steps to Freedom
22 Randall Road
Kenilworth
Warks CV8 1JY
Helpline: 01926 851608
10.00am–10.00pm daily

No Panic
93 Brands Farm Way
Randlay
Telford
Shropshire
Helpline: 01952 590545
10.00am–10.00pm daily

Phobic Action
Hornbeam House
Claybury Grounds
Woodford Green

Essex IG8 8PR
Admin tel: 0181 559 2551
Helpline: 0181 559 2459

Phobics Society
4 Cheltenham Road
Chorlton-cum-Hardy
Manchester M21 1QN
Tel: 0161 881 1937

Relaxation for Living
29 Burwood Park Road
Walton on Thames
Surrey KT12 5LH

Tranquillizers

CITA (Council for Involuntary
Tranquilliser Abuse)
Helpline: 0151 949 0102
10.00am–1.00pm Monday–Friday

Tranquillizer Anxiety Stress Help
Association (TASHA)
R Block, West Middlesex Hospital
Twickenham Road
Isleworth, Middlesex TW7 6AF
Admin tel: 0181 569 3333
Fax: 0181 568 0062
Helpline 0181 560 6601

Bereavement

CRUSE Bereavement Care
CRUSE House
126 Sheen Road
Richmond
Surrey TW9 1UR
Admin tel: 0181 940 4818
Fax: 0181 940 7638
Helpline: 0171 332 7227
Monday–Friday 9.30am–5.00pm
For local branches, see local telephone
book

Compassionate Friends (for bereaved
parents)
53 North Street
Bristol BS3 1EN
Tel: 0117 953 9639

Care Concern (for Jewish Women)
120 Oakley Road North
London N20
Tel: 0181 446 5418

Child Death Helpline
c/o Great Ormond Street Hospital
London WC1N 3JH
Helpline: 0800 282986

Cot Death Society
1 Browning Close
Thatcham
Berks RG13 4AU
Admin tel/fax: 01635 861 771

Foundation for the Study of Infant
Deaths (Cot Death)
14 Halkin Street
London SW1X 7DP
Admin tel: 0171 235 0965.
Fax: 0171 823 1986
Cot death helpline: 0171 235 1721

Lesbian and Gay Bereavement Project
The Unitarian Rooms
Hoop Lane
London NW11 8BF
Admin tel: 0181 200 0511
Helpline: 0181 455 8894
7.00pm–midnight daily

Miscarriage Association England
Clayton Hospital
Northgate
Wakefield, Yorks
Tel: 01924 200 799

Miscarriage Association Northern
Ireland
Ballykinler, nr Downpatrick
Tel: 01396 851596

Miscarriage Association Scotland
23 Castle Street
Edinburgh EH2 3DN
Admin tel/fax: 0131 220 3841
Helpline: 0131 334 8883

National Association of Bereavement
Services (NABS)
20 Norton Folgate

London E1 6DB
Admin tel/fax: 0171 247 0617
Referrals: 0171 247 1080

Society for Counselling and
Information on Miscarriage (SCIM)
12 Renfield Street
Glasgow G2 5AL
Admin tel/fax: 0141 221 1586

Stillbirth and Neonatal Death Society
(SANDS)
28 Portland Place
London W1N 4DE
Admin tel: 0171 436 7940
Fax: 0171 436 3715

Support Around Termination for
Abnormality (SATFA)
73 Charlotte Street
London W1P 1LB
Admin tel/fax: 0171 631 0280
Helpline: 0171 631 0285

Drug Addiction/Dependence

Drugline Ltd
9a Brockley Cross
London SE4 2AB
National helpline: 0181 692 4975
daily 9.00am–4.00pm except Tuesday
1.00pm–4.00pm

Freephone Drugline:
Dial 100 and ask operator for
Freephone Drugline

Families Anonymous
Doddington and Rollo Community
Association
Charlotte Despard Avenue
London SW11 5JE
Helpline: 0171 498 4680
Monday–Friday 1.00pm–4.30pm, plus
referral at weekends

Institute for Study of Drug
Dependence
Waterbridge House
32–36 Loman Street
London SE1 0EE
Admin tel: 0171 928 1211
Fax: 0171 928 1771

Narcotics Anonymous UK Service
Office
PO Box 1980
London N19 3LS
Admin tel: 0171 272 9040
Helpline: 0171 489 9005
10.00am–8.00pm daily

National Drugs Helpline
Network Scotland
The Mews
57 Ruthven Lane
Glasgow G12 9JQ
National helpline: 0800 776600
24 hours; foreign language service
details on request

Release
388 Old Street
London EC1V 9LT
Admin tel: 0171 729 5255.
Fax: 0171 729 2599
Helplines: 0171 729 9904
10.00am–6.00pm;
0171 603 8654 overnight
Drugs in schools line: 0345 366666
10.00am–6.00pm

Re-Solv Enquiries
30a High Street
Stone
Staffs ST15 8AW
Helpline: 01785 817 885
9.00am–5.00pm weekdays
(Enquiries regarding solvent abuse)

SCODA (Standing Conference on
Drug Abuse)
Waterbridge House
32–36 Loman Street
London SE1 0EE
Admin tel: 0171 928 9500
Fax: 0171 928 3343

Scottish Drugs Forum
Shaftesbury House
5 Waterloo Street
Glasgow G2 6AY

Admin tel: 0141 221 1175
Fax: 0141 248 6414

Family Stress

Alzheimers Disease Society
Gordon House
10 Greencoat Place
London SW1P 1PH
Admin tel: 0171 306 0606
Fax: 0171 306 0808
Helpline: 0171 306 0833

Carers National Association
20–25 Glasshouse Yard
London EC1A 4JS
Admin tel: 0171 490 8818
Fax: 0171 490 8824
Helpline: 0171 490 8898
Monday–Friday 7.30am–5.30pm

Catholic Marriage Advisory Council
Clitherow House
1 Blythe Mews
Blythe Road
London W14 0NW
Tel: 0171 371 1341

Childline
Freepost 1111
London N1 0BR
Helpline: 0800 1111
24 hour, nationwide

CRY-SIS Support Group
BM-CRYSIS
London WC1N 3XX
Helpline: 0171 404 5011
Daily 8.00am–11.00pm
(For support and advice to parents
whose babies cry incessantly, have
sleep problems, etc.)

Gingerbread
35 Wellington Street
London WC2E 7BN
Tel: 0171 240 0953 Fax: 0171 836 4500
For local groups please see local
phone book

Jewish Marriage Council
23 Ravenshurst Avenue
London NW4 4EE
Tel: 0181 203 6311
**24-hour helplines: for outside
London, 0345 581999;
London, 0181 203 6211**

National Council for Divorced and
Separated
13 High Street
Little Shelford
Cambridge CB2 5ES
Tel: 01533 708 880
See local phone book for branches
nationwide

National Council for One Parent
Families
255 Kentish Town Road
London NW5 2LX
Tel: 0171 267 1361 Fax: 0171 482 4851

National Family Mediation
9 Tavistock Place
London WC1H 9SN
Tel: 0171 383 5993 Fax: 0171 383 5994

Parents Anonymous (London)
6 Manor Gardens
London N7 6LA
Tel: 0181 263 8918
(For parents potentially or actually
involved in child abuse)

Relate – formerly Marriage Guidance
Council
Herbert Gray College
Little Church Street
Rugby
Warks CV21 3AP
Admin tel: 01788 573241
Fax: 01788 535007
For local centres, see local phone
book

Tavistock Institute of Marital Studies
Tavistock Centre

120 Belsize Lane
London NW3 5BA
Admin tel: 0171 435 7111
Fax: 0171 435 1080

Union of Muslim Organisations of
UK and Eire
109 Campden Hill Road
London W8 7TL
Admin tel: 0171 229 0538
(Offers marriage counselling
services)

Women's Aid Federation
(England) Ltd
PO Box 391
Bristol BS99 7WS
Admin tel: 0117 963 3494
Fax: 0117 942 1413
Mon–Friday 10.00am–1.00pm,
Tues/Wed/Thurs 2.00pm–4.00pm
Helpline: 0117 963 3542
10.30am–4.00pm, 7.30pm–10.00pm
daily

Others
**Benefits Agency Free Helpline:
English 0800 666555
Chinese 0800 252 451
Punjabi 0800 521 360
Urdu 0800 289 188
Welsh 0800 289 011**

British Association for Counselling
37a Sheep Street
Rugby
Warks CV21 3BX
Admin tel: 01788 550 899
Information line: 01788 578 328

British Wheel of Yoga
1 Hamilton Place
Boston Road
Sleaford
Lincs NG34 7ES
Tel: 0529 306851

Drug Information Centre
Pharmacy Department
Guy's Hospital
St Thomas Street
London SE1 9RT
Tel: 0171 378 0023

Health Service Ombudsman
England: 0171 217 4051
Scotland: 0131 225 7465
Wales: 01222 394621
Northern Ireland: 01232 233 812

National Retreat Association
Liddon House
24 South Audley Street
London W1Y 5DL
Tel/fax: 0171 493 3534

Pain Concern (UK)
PO Box 318
Canterbury
Kent CT4 5DP
Admin tel: 01227 832 103
Helpline: 01227 264677
(Support for all sufferers of chronic
pain and their carers)

Patients Association
PO Box 935
Harrow
Middlesex HA1 3YJ
Admin tel: 0181 423 9111
Fax: 0181 423 9119
Patients' helpline: 0181 423 8999
(Advice to individual patients and
carers on rights, complaints
procedures, access to health services
and self-help groups)

Transcendental Meditation (TM)
FREEPOST
London SW1P 4YY
Tel: 0800 269303
Fax: 01695 27499
(Tel: Freephone 0800 269 303)

Yoga for Health Foundation
Ickwell Bury
Biggleswade
Beds SG18 9EF
Tel: 01767 627271

INDEX